MOVE *freely*

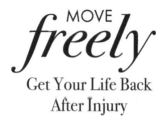

MOVE *freely*

Get Your Life Back
After Injury

HELEN M. BLAKE, MD

NEW YORK

LONDON • NASHVILLE • MELBOURNE • VANCOUVER

MOVE *freely*
Get Your Life Back After Injury

© 2020 HELEN M. BLAKE, MD

Published in New York, New York, by Morgan James Publishing in partnership with Difference Press. Morgan James is a trademark of Morgan James, LLC. www.MorganJamesPublishing.com

ISBN 978-1-64279-458-8   paperback

33614081568965

ISBN 978-1-64279-459-5   eBook
Library of Congress Control Number: 2019931795

Interior Design by:
Bonnie Bushman
The Whole Caboodle Graphic Design

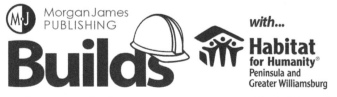

In an effort to support local communities, raise awareness and funds, Morgan James Publishing donates a percentage of all book sales for the life of each book to Habitat for Humanity Peninsula and Greater Williamsburg.

Get involved today! Visit
www.MorganJamesBuilds.com

For my patients:
Thank you for sharing your challenges with me.
Thank you for your trust in me.
You are my daily inspiration.

Table of Contents

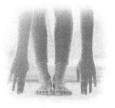

Chapter 1

You Are Not Your Pain

If you have opened this book, then you or a loved one is suffering from pain. You have come to the right place. I am here to help! As you know, pain is an overwhelming health problem within our society. Pain can present as a consequence of injury or disease. After our bodies have healed, pain often wonderfully lifts from our bodies and we are restored with barely a memory that it consumed us.

However, sometimes it lingers on, uncontrolled, and for seemingly no reason. We can try to fight it with strong medications, injections, surgeries, and therapy, but it persists, relentless in its destruction of our being. Pain can destroy careers and relationships, and sometimes pain robs us of our very will to live.

I wrote this book to help my patients realize that they have control over many aspects of their experience of pain and to lead them toward a lifestyle devoted to making targeted changes in their routine. This will improve their pain by decreasing the inflammation and stress in their bodies.

It's hard to survive and recover from an injury and realize that your body has been changed permanently. Our bodies and minds are our partners in life. We need both to be as healthy as possible so that we can pursue our dreams. When our bodies betray us and we are left with pain that effects our ability to function, we face many fears, frustrations, and obstacles in our pursuit of health.

I'm reminded of a teething infant. Can you imagine what we each go through just to erupt our teeth? If you have never had a toothache, I can assure you tooth pain is some of the worst pain out there. Imagine you are a small baby, who has only known love, cuddling, and pureed baby foods. You are stirred from sleep by a relentless throb in your mouth. You have never felt pain before. You don't know what is happening. So you cry, and cry, and cry. I imagine that in babies' innocent minds, they feel like that pain might never leave. They might fear that this pain will be their new normal.

Facing that idea is very scary. None of us intend to live our life in pain. None of us intend to have uncertainty about our ability to exist without pain. I have found in my practice of medicine, and my devotion to my patients who are suffering from pain, that the mind has an incredible way of taking control of how we experience the insults and injuries that occur to us in our lives.

What makes the difference between a person who sustains a terrible life-altering injury and goes back to work versus one who has a relatively minor injury yet never seems to be able to return to the demands of daily life? The unexpected can occur to any of us and in many ways. It could be the unexpected development of pain related to cancer, the diagnosis of a chronic illness like fibromyalgia or autoimmune disease-causing pain, an injury at work, or a car accident that you never expected. These moments occur during our lives, and these are circumstances over which we generally have no control. I don't think that any of us truly realize how our lives can change in one moment until it happens to us.

Most of the patients that I see in my practice have had long-standing pain. Most of them have suffered during their recovery from multiple surgeries, from the prescription of medications that don't serve them, and from physical therapy that they say has only hurt them.

Sometimes I see patients who are only beginning their partnership with pain. They have recently been injured at work or in an accident and, through no fault of their own, face changes to their lives and livelihoods that are unexpected and certainly undesired. When they first come to me, many of them feel helpless, hopeless, and fearful of what the future might bring.

As I strive to help these patients with medications, injections, interventions, and referrals for surgeries, my hope is that they get better. My hope for each of my patients is that I can help them thrive as the best version of themselves after the unexpected has occurred. My goal is to inspire them to rise up in the face of their pain.

So many times, I find that my patients' paths toward improvement are influenced by their own thoughts, emotions, and actions. People who choose the path of hope and direct their thoughts toward goals that serve to improve their lives have different outcomes than those who settle into despair or are seduced by the thought of settlements or disability pay.

In my training in pain management at New York's Weill Cornell Medical Center, I was able to care for many patients with many different causes of pain. I spent a year rotating through Memorial Sloan Kettering Cancer Hospital, serving the most complicated of cancer patients, and the Hospital for Special Surgery, serving those who are injured and recovering from orthopedic conditions. I had experiences and training that allowed me to present my patients with medical options to help change their experience with their pain. While these options are effective in many cases, as I've grown deeper in my experience and my engagement with my patients in private practice, I've realized that the difference between success and failure comes from something much deeper and much more driven by the relationship I form with patients themselves. It comes from a relationship that unfortunately in today's medical world is difficult to achieve in a traditional clinical environment.

Due to the time limitations that many physicians have in short patient visits, that relationship is compromised and less effective than it could be. I take the time that I can with each new patient I see to truly try to understand the many different elements of their pain. I want to understand each patient's motivation, their home life, their sleep habits, their nutrition, and their general outlook on their pain.

I devote time to coaching them through some of their most difficult obstacles in managing their life in pain. I try to help patients change the way that they see the world after their pain. After all, their world hasn't changed after their injury, their dreams haven't changed, and the love they have around them hasn't changed. The only thing that has changed is the circumstances. They now have a new villain in their life: Pain. There are so many solutions for patients who are suffering from pain, but some of the most effective strategies are simple ones that we can engage in our lives without the help of a medication, surgery, or injection. These strategies capitalize on the strength that we have within ourselves and the motivation we have to move forward in our lives. The most amazing results come through not allowing the pain that you experience to keep you down.

You are not your pain. You are the same person you were before you were injured; you have the same aspirations, goals, obligations, and opportunities. The moment that you allow your pain to start limiting your experience with life is the moment that you stop living the life you choose.

I seek to truly get to know and love my patients and help them see a path forward. I can't promise any miracles. Unfortunately, there are some conditions for which even the cleverest of doctors and interventions or most cutting-edge therapies won't serve to fully end patients' suffering. However, even in these seemingly hopeless cases, I can change your experience with your pain and give you some hope. That is what my true passion and calling is—to help you end your suffering.

I wrote this book for you, my reader, my patient. I wrote this book for you who may struggle with the limitations that have been set before you in your life due to the pain and injury that you've experienced. I want to give you hope that there is light at the end of this tunnel.

You may feel limited at this moment in your life. You may feel as though just getting out of bed is too much for you to bear. I will show you a way to manage your pain systematically with simple changes in your routine

You can get your life back. You will move freely again. You are able to live, breathe, think, and love. With these vital faculties you can set your mind on a goal before you. You will rise above this experience of pain.

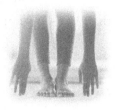

Chapter 2

You Are Not Alone

Y ou are not alone. I am here to help you. I have devoted my life and my career to you. You may come to me fresh from injury and new to the realization that pain is a part of your life. You may come to me after you have already spent years in treatment for your pain. You might be challenged with low expectations set by negative experiences you have had with other doctors. You may have encountered medical professionals who have tried to tell you that your pain is not real.

Patients come to me with appalling stories about how they were treated by other doctors, therapists, and surgeons whom they have encountered on their journey. I have heard stories of people being put down and made to feel guilty for the pain they experience. Patients have been told that their pain was permanent, that their only hope was to continuously rely on strong medications, that they could never work again, and that they would have to give up the activities that give them joy. I have had patients tell me their former doctor said, "You will be like this the rest of your life; get used to it."

Have you had interactions such as these? Is that your story? How do these interactions serve you, my patient? These interactions limit you. If you choose to make these horror stories, this ill-given "advice" your treatment plan, I assure you, the pain will only persist.

I have helped many patients on a pathway to the other side of their pain. Some of these patients have been injured in motor vehicle accidents. Some have been facing life-threatening diagnoses, like cancer, or chronic diagnoses, like fibromyalgia. Some have been injured at work and have their very livelihood at stake if their pain remains uncontrolled. Some have just had a simple knee surgery and developed pain after surgery out of proportion to what other patients usually experience.

You may have been told that you are at fault for the pain and that there is something wrong with you or your coping mechanisms. You may have been prescribed strong medications after surgery like hydrocodone, dutifully followed the directions on the bottle that state, "Take one pill every four hours for pain," and, after requesting refill for the medication a few times, been accused of inappropriate use by your doctor of the medications when you were suffering from pain that was still out of control.

Perhaps you had a truly empathetic and compassionate doctor who prescribed a medication that didn't serve you, and on each return visit, your wonderful doctor increased your medication even though there was no real sign that it was working for you. After months or even years on the medication, your pain is still not improved and you have side effects that are limiting you and making you nearly as uncomfortable as the pain itself.

If this is your past, I am sorry. I have seen each of these stories in my practice. I have helped each of these patients redesign their future.

The history and past experiences of patients when they first come to see me is always reflected in their experience of pain now. Many patients are very focused on the past. They describe anger toward the person who injured them in an accident, they describe frustration with the system of worker's compensation if they have been injured at work, or they express despair about the circumstances of their diagnosis with chronic conditions. Patients often tell stories of their past, and in retelling their history, they relive the assault that the process of their injury created. However, when I can help patients see that it's not their past but their future that matters, amazing changes start to happen.

I recall a patient of mine who was suffering from terminal breast cancer. She was thirty-six years old and had merely months to live. Her outlook and acceptance of her terminal destiny was amazing. She was facing death, but despite that circumstance, her outlook was resolute to get everything possible out of the time that she had left. She shared with me that one of the biggest tragedies in her life was the pain that she felt when her three-year-old child made her giggle because the pain in her chest wall from the tumors that were pressing on her nerves had become so severe. Here this woman sat before me, facing death, and mourning the fact that the simple pleasure of joyfully laughing with her child was no longer available to her.

We implanted in her a device that gave her medication directly into her spinal fluid, and that effectively eliminated her pain. When she awoke from the anesthesia in the recovery room, her family surrounded her. There, in the recovery room, a miracle happened. Her sweet, beautiful, and boisterous three-year-old made her laugh. For the first time in months, she was able to laugh with her child without pain.

There are no words in the English language to describe the joy that spread over her face. There is no word that adequately relates the profound feeling of love, relief, and happiness that was in that room that day. Ella (all names changed for the patients' privacy) died from her cancer three months later. However, she died with the memories of her and her family's laughter in her heart.

It is the profound privilege of being part of these small miracles that motivates me to devote my career to minimizing patients' suffering.

What Will Your Miracle Be?

Most miracles that I witness are not quite as dramatic as Ella's, but a miracle is born every time I help a patient conquer their greatest challenge created by their pain condition.

James, an executive of a large national corporation, came to me with disabling knee pain after an injury that had occurred years prior. As a youth, he'd injured himself while playing team sports. Somewhere along the line, he became reliant on opiate medications to control the pain. Despite never before seeing a pain management doctor, he was taking unusually high doses of very strong pain medications. James came to see me because his primary doctor had decided that he no longer felt comfortable prescribing to James. James felt discarded by his family doctor. He stated, "I always took the medications the way he prescribed them; I don't know what I did wrong. I don't understand why he won't prescribe my medicine to me anymore."

To say James was reluctant to see me for the first time is an understatement. When we first met, he was scared that I might strip his medications away from him, torture him with the symptoms of withdrawal, and then discharge him unceremoniously into the world with no way to manage his pain.

I suppose he had reason for fear. Increasingly, in this current era of Centers for Disease Control-guided opiate prescription recommendations, many family physicians who have previously offered their patients opioid medications are discontinuing them suddenly or referring patients to specialists like me to manage or wean them off their medications. Patients often don't realize that specialists can lead them to other options to manage their pain. These options can range from other medications, interventions, or therapies that are actually more effective at treating their condition and improving their pain.

Under my care, James did indeed wean completely from his opiates. Be assured, I didn't force him to do that. He came off his medications driven by his own will. He took power over his thoughts, and I dove into the effective use of medications that actually improved his condition. He made subtle changes in his life that created a profound impact on his circumstances.

When James first came to see me, he was reliant on a type of pain management patch that he changed every three days. When he placed these patches on his sensitive skin they created burns. *His medication burned his skin!* He was so desperate for pain relief that he dutifully reapplied and changed his pain patches every three days for more than two years, believing that the treatment his doctor had given him was the best choice for him. Despite the fact that his medication was actually causing him harm, he believed that he was in the best condition he would ever be.

He never actually experienced an improvement of his pain symptoms.

When patients first come to see me, they complete a comprehensive questionnaire that I review before meeting them. When James first came to see me, he described his pain as "the worst pain imaginable" despite his use of fentanyl patches. "I guess they make the pain more tolerable," he said to me, "but really, the pain is still powerfully there."

I have similar conversations with patients all the time. Patients come to me on medications that are creating side effects that are actually limiting their lives, and the medications aren't even serving the purpose of making large improvements on their pain.

In any other form of medicine, if you were taking a medication that was not improving your diagnosis and causing major side effects (like burning your skin), you would stop taking it. Patients with pain are different. Patients suffering from pain come to me feeling that their medications are the only thing that gives them hope. For some people, their medications are the only thing that makes life livable for them.

The burning skin wasn't his only side effect. James, through the course of his employment, had to walk long distances on the business property. His fentanyl and the narcotic medications would make him sweat profusely. He stated that he would entertain visiting executives and his company leadership and he would be embarrassed by how profusely he would sweat while making presentations or merely leading them around the property.

James had developed crushing anxiety during these visits, and he felt limited in his ability for further career advancement. He feared being accused of poor performance and losing his job. He was considering filing for permanent disability. Additionally, he couldn't pleasure his wife anymore, due to the side effects of the medications. He felt devoid of any basic human pleasure.

After educating him on the ways that the side effects he was experiencing from his medication, rather than his orthopedic condition, were limiting his lifestyle, we started decreasing his pain medication and started implementing treatment for his anxiety. He practiced many of the strategies I outline in this book and started a dialog of positive self-talk. He developed a new acceptance of the condition that he had.

The remarkable thing is that his pain started improving despite his taking less medication. He started taking care of himself; he started exercising. He started engaging in team sports, and his social life flourished. His relationships started improving. When I first met James, he was on the brink of divorce from his spouse, but with his strategic commitment to a process that improved not only his pain but also the entire circumstances around him, the marriage was invigorated. He became stronger and more ready to conquer life and achieve his dreams.

Love Thy Neighbor, but Don't Forget to Love Thyself
Another patient, Jessica, first came to see me at the end of her career. She had suffered from fibromyalgia for years and had limiting side effects from any medications that doctors provided to her. She had chosen to live her life without medication for her pain.

She was depressed, anxious, and had many health problems, ranging from high blood pressure and type 2 diabetes to autoimmune dysfunction. When she first submitted her new patient paperwork, she had to use three pages just to outline all the medications that she was on to manage her health conditions.

In the first few visits with her, I spent time talking and exploring elements of her lifestyle with her. I found that even though she had a career as a nurse, she took horrible care of herself. She was also the mother of eight grown children and had a total of twenty-four grandchildren who lived in the area. While working full time as a nurse, she also took care of her grandchildren in her spare time. She devoted an enormous amount of energy to them. Yet she couldn't find the energy to prepare herself a single healthy meal per day. She was overweight, tired, depressed, and fatigued. She stated that at work she brought a bottle of Coca-Cola or lemonade and would subsist on goldfish crackers and other inexpensive cookies and snacks. She justified this because she spent a significant amount of money supporting her children's families. She also ate fast food once per day because she frequently left directly from her night shift as a nurse to care for her grandchildren to help save her children on the cost of childcare.

She was completely perplexed and frustrated about why her medical conditions were not improving with escalating diabetes and high blood pressure medications. She felt out of control and hopeless. When she started changing her diet and putting her needs before her adult children's, her health started changing.

She started following a strategic meal plan that worked toward decreasing inflammation. She found not only that her pain started to improve but also that all her chronic conditions started to lift.

Her eczema, which she had suffered since childhood, improved substantially. Her asthma, for which she initially required three medications to control, came to require only an occasional rescue inhaler. Her diabetes, for which she was on two different types of insulin as well as an oral anti-diabetic medication, went into complete remission. She lost sixty pounds, and she emerged at the age of sixty, after working with me for just over a year, with a whole new outlook on life. She not only was prepared to thrive through the last five years of her nursing career before retirement but also found greater satisfaction in all her relationships. She found that when she spent time loving herself, all her family members rose up in support around her.

I am also reminded of Jerry. Jerry was injured at work. He fractured one of the vertebral bodies in his spine when he fell from a ladder. He required emergency spinal surgery to stabilize his spine. As he was rushed to surgery, he was losing the feeling in his legs and was incontinent, losing control of both urine and stool. He feared in that very moment that his life was never going to be the same.

He was correct. After surgery, his recovery was complicated by infections, and he had to have two more operations to manage the consequences of the infections. His surgeon compassionately prescribed him pain medication to manage the pain surrounding his surgeries. But even after surgery, he suffered from severe pain. His doctor kept increasing his pain medications. When he first came to me, he was taking more than 300 milligrams' equivalent of morphine per day.

He was depressed. He hadn't worked in seven years. He had developed what is called urinary retention, which can be a side effect of opioid medications. He required medication to help him with the basic bodily function of urination. He was severely constipated, which is also a potential side effect of opiates. He took three different daily medications to treat his constipation and also needed weekly enemas to provoke bowel movements. He had developed impotence, also a side effect of the medications. He tried three different medications to help provoke erections, but none were successful. He had not had sex with his wife in three years.

In addition to the limitations placed on his bodily functions because of his medication, he couldn't participate in activities that gave him great joy. He formerly took great pride in the landscaping of his home, but even with the medication at such a high dose, merely ten minutes outside would send him to the couch for weeks.

Depressed and despondent, he stated clearly, "I don't know if these medications are working for me, but they're the only thing that I have."

Jerry was reliant on these medications. Medications that weren't even working to control his pain. At this point, he was literally losing everything around him in his life, even his basic bodily functions.

No doctor had ever before spent the time to counsel Jerry on how all of these symptoms were a consequence of the medication he was taking. In his mind, no one had any idea why these conditions were happening to him. His thoughts told him that he had terrible luck.

He became motivated to change his life by weaning off all his medications. Four months into our journey together, he had stopped using opiate medications and no longer required the medications for his constipation, urinary retention, and impotence. His entire life around him improved. He grew to accept the limitations that his body had after his injury. Unfortunately, due to the nature of his injuries and the fact that he had already been out of work for seven years prior to meeting me, he may never work traditionally again. However, he has started volunteering with his church delivering meals to the elderly and walking pets for a local humane society.

He has a completely new outlook on life and contributes to the world around him in a more meaningful way than he had been able to while on medication.

Each of my patients inspire me on a daily basis with the small miracles. Each small success reinforces to them that small changes work and motivates them toward a better life for themselves.

Impossible pain conditions are possible to overcome. How do we do it together? We work through a program that has its roots in a variety of fields of research. Each of the elements of this plan has been shown to be superior to medications in the improvement of pain scores. This plan will lead you through seven simple changes to the way that you think and process the information around us.

You can create amazing changes in your life. Come follow me.

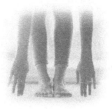

Chapter 3

Do What It Takes

While the elements of this program are very simple, I can't claim that this program is easy. It takes commitment to meet your goals. It requires trusting the process when perhaps you have lost your capacity to trust the medical community a long time ago. This process will require allowing yourself to feel some discomfort. I promise that the reward is worth it. The changes that you can make in your life are unbelievable.

Changing your circumstances requires massive action. It doesn't happen overnight. It will take a commitment to the plan over a period of days, weeks, months, and years. With each day that you make the commitment to change you are moving closer toward your goals. This process is not just about the management of pain. This process is about making improvements that will change your entire life.

There is no new magic in this program. Even if these concepts are new to you, most of these concepts are well described and backed by research that has demonstrated their impact on people's pain scores. I assure you that this program, when applied to any condition, can lead you toward positive change in your life. The hardest part is establishing the routine for change.

You are here to feel better. Regardless of your current circumstances, this program will help you to feel better. When you consistently create and follow a routine that implements the steps that I outline below, you will realize dramatic changes in your life.

This process will renew your life with new energy and new ways of thinking about your circumstances. As you renew your life and focus on your nutrition, activity level, and relationship with yourself, you will find that how you feel about the circumstances that your injury and pain condition has created for you can be changed.

There are seven steps to this model. Together they will *renew* you and effect positive change in your life.

The first step is to rise up! You will address the power of your mind and how the thoughts that you choose to believe are more powerful than anything external to you. You will learn a different way to manage the negative thoughts and feelings that you may experience through your painful condition. You will find how small changes in your thoughts can change the way that you're showing up to your relationships, to your job, to your physicians, and to your family. As we work to reframe the negative thoughts that might limit you, you will find the power to rise above your pain and take the next steps forward.

The second step is to eat to end inflammation. In this chapter, we will address the powerful benefit of an anti-inflammatory diet. We will outline the different foods that you might be able to eat that will create positive impact on your body and mind. With proper nourishment, you will find your pain will improve through decreasing the inflammation at its source.

After we learn how to nourish your body, we will explore ways to nourish your mind. In this chapter, we will discuss the art of meditation and mindfulness and how a simple regular practice of mindfulness can create impact toward improving your pain. Not only will your pain scores improve, but your stress levels will drop, your likelihood to react negatively to circumstances around you will decrease, and your sleep will improve. Mindfulness and meditation can improve the quality of your life and your coping abilities.

We will then dive into the profound fear of movement many of my patients have developed and learn how to exercise freely. When you allow yourself to become sedentary due to your pain, you become increasingly deconditioned. We must build back our physical abilities when we have been sedentary for a period of time. I will give you some simple exercises that will strengthen your core and increase your flexibility. This will help you to move more freely despite your pain and better face the challenges of your day.

Chapter 8 will explore how work matters. We will discuss your profession, your career, and your goals. We will address the powerful impact that continuing on the path of reaching your professional goals and explore the financial security that work brings and its impact on your mindset. Is your body no longer able to do the job you once loved? We will also address options you might have to move forward and move into a different career where you could find satisfaction.

Walk into any drugstore and ask for a supplement to help with your pain, and you will be presented with so many options it's mind boggling. In chapter 9, we will learn about supplements for success and discuss holistic and natural options that are widely available to improve your pain.

We will also explore some of the most common minimally invasive therapies your doctor may discuss with you to address your pain symptoms. We will talk about what the purpose of these therapies are and what role they might play in the management of your pain.

Finally, we will explore ways that you can address your greatest obstacles. Let's face it, obstacles are inevitable. We can conquer them together and create a clear path forward.

No matter how independent you might be, assembling the right team around you is important. We will discuss how choosing the right physician, psychologist, physical therapist, or coach is at the core of your success. I will help you create a support network around you that will help you implement the changes that we address in this book to make the greatest progress in your pain.

We can do this! You can improve you pain and move freely again. Let's do it together!

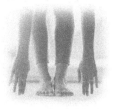

Chapter 4

Rise Up!

O ur minds have an incredible capacity to think. In fact, we have nearly seventy thousand thoughts per day, and an average of fifty thoughts per waking minute. Our thoughts have the incredible power to help us grow, create our goals, keep our families safe, and plan our days. There is nothing you have ever done that hasn't been initiated by a thought in your mind.

Despite the power of your thoughts, most of us are completely unaware of the quantity and quality of the thoughts in our mind. Most of us are completely unaware of how managing the quality of our thoughts can create improvements in our life. If more of us learned to recognize the thoughts that we are having and worked to change negative thought patterns to more positive ones, I assure you the world would be a much better place. I won't try to tackle the world in this book, but I hope to inspire you to become more aware of your thoughts and how some changes in your thought patterns can create changes in your life.

Every thought that we have creates an emotion within us. These emotions influence our actions. They influence how we show up in our relationships, our jobs, and for ourselves.

I am not trying to suggest that your pain is in your mind. However, I promise you that your mind has the incredible capacity to control your pain. Human beings have an immense ability to use their thoughts to create their perceptions of the world around them.

A pivotal research study performed in 2015 at the Colorado University in Boulder looked at three different ways of thinking to understand the way people's thoughts can influence pain processing in the brain. They used advanced imaging called functional magnetic resonance imaging to study participants when painful heat was applied to their arms. Researchers performed scans on these participants under three different conditions:

1. The first group of participants were asked to not think of anything in particular while being subjected to the painful heat.
2. The second group of participants were asked to imagine that the burning heat was actually causing irreparable damage to their skin.
3. The third group of participants were asked to imagine that this burning heat was actually a very welcome pleasant sensation on an extremely cold day.

Guess what? In all three cases the temperature of the heat was identical, but the people who imagined the heat was a welcome and pleasant sensation described a lower overall pain score. The people who were told to imagine that the sensation of burning was causing irreparable damage could hardly tolerate completing the study. When the participant's brains were scanned the researchers found two different pathways where pain information was processed. One pathway was for experiencing the physical pain. The images were identical in all three of the conditions. However, they noticed a second brain pathway that changed in intensity depending on the type of thoughts the participant was told to create. This pathway was more related to the emotional component of the pain and changed significantly between the three groups. This pathway was found to be more closely related to the pain score that the patients identified rather than the actual physical sensation.

This study shows the power of "cognitive self-regulation" in the world of pain management. It shows that what you think can have a profound impact on how you feel.

Are there any times in your life that you can think of where you've been able to change your perspective on a painful situation to make it seem more agreeable? If you were an athlete were there ever opportunities where you "pushed through" the pain to achieve an unimaginable goal? When we direct energy toward a goal, we are capable of remarkable things. I want to introduce you to a few examples of how people reframe their thoughts toward a more positive alternative and can improve their experience as they conquer difficult circumstances.

The Resilience of a Soldier Is in All of Us

Has anyone in your life served in the armed forces? When soldiers are called to duty and join basic training, their bodies are subjected to rigorous conditioning so that they can meet the physical demands of combat. Can you imagine the physical pain when they first start basic training? Can you imagine the emotional challenges they face in combat, facing potential injury to their bodies or even death? Whenever we move our bodies outside of our comfort zone there is often a bit of discomfort involved. Discomfort is a part of life, but so is the joy of winning the fight. A soldier learns to focus on the glory of victory, rather than the discomfort of the process.

This is a learned skill. This skill can be developed in all of us. We send soldiers to basic training because no one can face the challenges of combat and expect to be successful without preparation and training. We learn how to be resilient. You need training to become resilient and face adversity. Just as soldiers can train their minds to face combat, you can train your mind to be better prepared to face your pain.

Laboring for Love

Childbirth is generally recognized as one of the most painful experiences a person can endure. Yet women all over the world choose to pursue the opportunity to bring children into the world. Despite the knowledge that they will endure unbelievable suffering in order to deliver their child, they joyfully attend doctor's visits and decorate nurseries excited to bring new life into their families. Can you imagine if women focused on the pain instead of the potential for the great reward of the love of a child? Why would anyone put themselves through that? How could anyone bear to procreate? Pregnant women instead usually choose to focus on the lovely things associated with childbirth. They focus on the idea of holding their infant child in their arms, they revel in the tiny clothing on display at baby stores, and they indulge in the love and support of their friends and family through baby showers. Without directing their thoughts to the positive aspects of childbirth, it would be so much more difficult to manage the challenges they face.

I assure you, just as the pregnant woman can direct her attention away from the certain pain and discomfort associated with childbirth, so can you learn to redirect your attention toward the positive aspects of your life and relationships. This instinctual ability we have to isolate one's negative thoughts and fears can be just as effective for you as it can be for women throughout the world when you learn to strengthen and develop it.

The Lies We Tell Ourselves

It is no secret that because of our culture, we have the tendency to accumulate an abundance of things. Yet many of us find ourselves assessing our closets and thinking "I have nothing to wear." We convince ourselves that we need all the gadgets cramming our kitchen drawers. Our homes are cluttered with magazines and knick-knacks. Our garages are full of tools that we used a single time.

Often we hold on to these things because we have invested money or time in them. Even though the money has been spent and the items have fulfilled their intended use, we hold on to them. This is often out of the guilt that we have about "wasting" whatever resource you have spent. This psychological phenomenon is what makes change so hard sometimes.

We have the tendency to continue things when we have invested time or money into them. There is no limit to what we will continue or hold on to. People hold on to clothes that have long been out of style. People continue bad marriages even when their physical or emotional health is at risk. People eat every last bit of food that was prepared by a loved one even when they are no longer hungry.

You may have been continuing medications or treatment plans that aren't really working. You can change this irrational pattern. You can conquer the guilt. The answer is in managing your thoughts.

Our brains are incredibly powerful. The thoughts that we create in our minds change our emotions, our perceptions, and our actions surrounding everything we do. This is such a powerful concept, but people are often resistant and hesitant to accept that their thoughts have the power to change their circumstances.

This is certainly not an immediate link. You can't think "I'm going to be a millionaire" and then instantly become one without some persistence and work. However, you can think and decide, "I have the ability and capacity to do the work needed to create my financial goals" and get a lot closer to becoming a millionaire than you are right now, even if you never actually achieve seven figures in your bank account.

My Pain Does Not Limit Me

Your thoughts are not limited by your pain. You can think whatever thoughts you choose to. Do you choose to create positive thoughts? Or do you choose negative thoughts? Will you choose to grow despite your circumstance of pain, or will you choose to allow your circumstances to become more desperate than they might be right now?

As you create positive thoughts around your pain, rather than focus on the fears that you might associate with your experience of pain, you can have powerful impacts on your body, your mind, and your life.

Your body is achieving miracles every day that it exists; your pain does not limit the miracles that your body can create. When suffering from chronic pain, many of you might struggle to find positive things to say about your body and your health. Positivity may be a challenge to create, but when you make small shifts in your thinking, you can change your emotion and perception of your pain.

Your mind and your body are not two separate entities. Every thought that processes through your mind is translated in some way to your body. When you say negative things to yourself about your condition, your medical care, your employer, or about any of your circumstances, you engage in a stream of negative thoughts. This is going to create a negative impact on your experience of your current circumstances.

If you think to yourself, "I'll never recover from this injury" or fear that the pain that you're experiencing is creating more damage to your body, you may find that your pain is more difficult to improve.

No one is immune from the possibility of entertaining negativity in their mindset when dealing with chronic pain. Suffering from pain stinks.

When you change your perspective dramatic and extraordinary things will happen to you.

When you think thoughts that do not serve you—like, "I can only function with medication"—you are giving that medication incredible power over your life. Does the medication deserve that power?

Let's go over this again, because I feel it warrants repeating. Every day, we are each creating numerous thoughts. You might, for example, think that for your particular pain mindset alone could not possibly help improve your condition. OK, I am not suggesting that your physical condition will improve. If you need surgery for a torn rotator cuff or a herniated disc, no amount of thought management will change that circumstance. However, your mindset can also have an impact on how well medications, surgery, or other treatments might work for you.

If you consistently create a pattern of thought where you are expecting the worst pain, or if you allow yourself to feel helpless about your pain, ruminate about the risks of surgery or the side effects of your medications, or focus on the limitations that you have because of pain, then you will surely put obstacles in your path, and you will experience greater pain intensity. You will likely require more medications and you will have less of an effect from treatments aimed at relieving your pain. You will be more likely never to return to work and become disabled from your pain. This negative pain mindset delays your recovery and predicts the development of pain that becomes chronic and constant.

You were born with the skills to be motivated to escape the pain. You just have to train yourself to use them. Think about when you've accidentally touched a hot stove. Your body and your mind are intimately connected and your hand will reflexively withdraw from that stimulus to keep you safe. You can learn to train your brain away from pain and create lasting improvements.

If you wake up every day and put yourself in a state where you are thinking about the limitations your pain is placing in your life, you will surely become limited by your pain.

Let's review: your thoughts create your emotions, which drive your actions, which change your circumstances.

What are some of your thoughts?

Here is a thought exercise based on one thought my patients have shared with me and how we have helped them reframe their thinking to create change:

I will never recover from this injury / I have the capacity to recover from this injury / I hope I will recover from this injury / I will recover from this injury.

Each of these statements is very similar.

Which statement do you identify with right now? Which statement do you see the possibility that you could agree with?

When you consider each of these thoughts, which thought makes you feel happy, uplifted, and hopeful for the future? Which thought brings you deeper into a state of despair?

Can you see that each thought creates a different emotion within you?

Perhaps you're not quite at the point where you're ready to say confidently, "I will recover from this injury," but perhaps you can focus on the statement "I have the capacity to recover from this injury." I promise you, that statement is true.

These thoughts create emotions. We choose to feel certain emotions. We allow our thoughts to create our emotions. Right now you might feel anger, frustration, despair, or hopelessness when you think of the limitations that are imposed on you by the experience of your pain. Consider if you instead retrain your brain to focus on thoughts that create positive emotions, such as hope, happiness, peace, growth, and acceptance. You will likely find that the way that you show up for yourself each day and the way that you approach your daily tasks will start to improve.

These strategies don't only have implications in the management of pain. These strategies can have implications in other arenas in your life where you find yourself coming short of your aspirations. These strategies can help you lose weight, achieve professional satisfaction, or conquer alcoholism and substance abuse, among many others. All these conditions are similar in that we create a negative distortion of our environments that perpetuates perceptions that do not serve us. When your perception differs from reality, you can be led toward health concerns such as depression and anxiety. Not only that, but these thought patterns also don't help you achieve your next raise!

Negative thoughts cause real damage to your relationships and to your experience of life. The longer you let these negative feelings and these negative thoughts influence your emotions and actions, the worse your circumstances will become.

Take control! You have the power! If you can follow simple steps to transition negative thoughts into positive, more rational, and productive thoughts, you will find that your experiences in your life only change for the better.

During each day, I encourage you to reflect and focus on all the good around you in your life.

Are you having trouble finding it?

Did you wake up this morning and breathe fresh air into your lungs? Be thankful for that; that is good.

Take a moment to reflect on the simple pleasures in life. These might be a soft carpet on your feet when you stepped out of bed or the joyful smile on your child's face when they first see you in the morning or the warm water you feel on your back during your shower. Reflect on the simple pleasures that bring you joy in your life. Reflect on the positive emotions you feel during these times. Most importantly, get a journal and write them down.

Each day, I want you to write down three things you are grateful to have or experience. These three things can be the same each day, or they can change from day to day. These are your anchors. In the moments when you struggle with negative thoughts, pull out your journal and read them to yourself. Focus on the positive emotions these thoughts evoke.

Don't worry, these exercises aren't all sunshine and roses. You can't make real growth unless you face your negative thoughts head on. Each day, I want you to spend ten minutes writing down whatever negative thoughts come to your mind. Some days, there may be many, and some days, there may be few. I want you to dive into these thoughts. How do they make you feel? What emotion do they create for you? How do you think each thought influences your actions and interactions with other people?

How do you want to feel instead? What thought would create that emotion? How would that change the way you show up? Each day, pick one thought to apply this exercise.

Example:

Initial Thought: "I will never be out of pain."

Emotion: frustrated, sad, depressed

Revised Thought: "I can make changes today that might improve my pain."

Emotion: hopeful, proud, determined, committed

How do you think the person with the revised thought shows up in his world compared to the initial thought? Who is more likely to make changes to improve their pain?

Create a Routine

One of the most important first steps in improving your mindset around your pain is to keep and maintain a healthy routine. For those of you who are recovering from an injury or are off work due to an injury or while recovering from surgery, you may not have a regular routine or obligations. A routine is particularly important in your case.

A routine must, at a minimum, include a consistent time each morning to awaken, consistent meal times, time for movement, time for mindfulness or meditation, and a consistent bedtime. I find that part of maintaining a healthy mindset is creating these simple routines. Without routine and structure in your life, it is all too easy to invite negative thoughts that do not serve you in the time you have left unstructured.

Setting a schedule, and then consistently showing up for your own self-imposed obligations, however mundane, is a powerful tool to create progress.

1. On a sheet of paper, or on a page in your journal, write today's date

2. Write the hours from 6:00 a.m. to 11:00 p.m. in thirty-minute increments

3. Write in any external obligations, such as doctor's appointments, therapy requirements, family obligations, and so on.

4. Decide on an appropriate bedtime and a time for waking in the morning. These times should be at least seven and not more than ten hours apart. I recommend the times of 7:00 a.m. and 11:00 p.m. The specific times can be adjusted to the needs of you and your family.

5. Place on the schedule the times that you will eat three meals.

6. Plan for thirty minutes of physical activity. We will discuss options for physical activity in a later chapter, but at the very least use this time to do gentle movements of the unaffected parts of your body or any exercises your physical therapist has encouraged you to do at home.

7. Plan for fifteen to thirty minutes to actively manage your thoughts and complete the thought exercises in this chapter.

8. Plan for at least fifty to thirty minutes of mindfulness or meditation. We will discuss how to practice this in a later chapter.

The rest of your time can be spent doing things that you enjoy, keeping your home in order or spending time with your support system and the people who make a positive impact to your life. The more time we spend with people and on things that serve us and the more we eliminate the people and thoughts that do not serve us, the more we will find positive movement toward our goal of improving our pain.

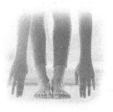

Chapter 5

Eat to End Inflammation

"What are the side effects of this medication, Doctor?" This is a daily question in my medical office. The same person who asks, "Will this medication cause me to gain weight?" often has no appreciation of how what she eats can have a profound influence in not just weight gain but also her experience of her pain condition by influencing the amount of inflammation in her body.

Any patient that requires a medication to control their pain would benefit also from following a "Pain Control" diet. A healthy diet can not only improve a person's overall health but also decrease the amount of pain-causing inflammation in the body and decreasing inflammation in the brain which results in less depression and fatigue.

It has never been clearer that the quality of the food we eat has a profound influence on our health. However, it seems as our knowledge has grown, so has confusion about what advice to follow for the best results. There are so many different books to read, plans to follow, and supplements to buy that it is easier sometimes to just ignore it all and settle in with our same old habits.

American diets have been increasingly focused on high-carbohydrate and processed foods that do not serve the human body. What we eat, and the macronutrient make-up of the meals we prepare can significantly influence the way we feel throughout the day. There is evidence that eating a low sugar, moderate protein, moderate healthy fat diet can actually decrease people's perception of pain and control anxiety and depression, resulting in people needing less medication to manage these chronic conditions.

Have you ever noticed after Thanksgiving dinner you get tired and sleepy? I have always heard people say that sleepiness was because of the amino acid tryptophan in the turkey that induces sleep. It is true that turkey has a high level of tryptophan that is converted to a neurotransmitter named serotonin and ultimately to the chemical melatonin in your brain, but if turkey was the only reason, then turkey

sandwiches would be inducing afternoon sleep in school children all over the country. What is so special about Thanksgiving is the volume of food we eat, specifically the volume of *carbohydrates*. Think about it. The "classic" American Thanksgiving plate is loaded with carbohydrates: mashed potatoes, sweet potatoes, corn casserole, stuffing, and rolls. Then we finish off the meal with a thick slice (or several slices) of pie—apple, pumpkin, pecan. I would venture to guess that most of you only end up with room on your plate for a meager two-ounce slice of turkey—hardly enough to blame the turkey's tryptophan on your sluggish afternoon.

What happens to you after you eat all those carbs? Your insulin levels shoot through the roof. After that spike, your blood sugar naturally drops significantly, and that drop in blood sugar triggers your sleepiness. Think back to last Thanksgiving: after the meal and the cleanup, when you finally were able to sit down on the couch with your family and watch football or movies or play a board game—how did you feel when you stood up after sitting for a while? Nearly universally, people feel achy and stiff after a big meal like Thanksgiving dinner. What's to blame? Carbohydrates that trigger inflammation in the body.

Can you reflect on your diet for the last three days? Which of the following foods have you been eating?

___Cereal   ___Shrimp   ___Bacon

___Salad   ___Spinach   ___Sausage

___Eggs   ___Lettuce   ___Potatoes

___Fish   ___Broccoli   ___Carrots

___Milk   ___Cookies   ___Corn

___Sugar   ___Cake   ___Green Beans

___Cream   ___Ice Cream   ___Peas

___Beef   ___Yogurt   ___Crackers

___Pork   ___Cottage Cheese   ___Cheese

___Chicken   ___Nuts   ___Spaghetti / Pasta

___Brussels Sprouts ___Chocolate   ___Tomatoes

___Candy   ___Chips   ___Avocado

___Noodles   ___Hamburgers   ___Salami / Bologna

___Bread   ___Hot Dots   ___Bagels

___Melon   ___Squash   ___Ice Cream

___Cauliflower   ___French Fries   ___Berries

___Apple   ___Lamb   ___Doughnuts

___Pear   ___Tortillas   ___Rolls

___Pastry   ___Whiskey   ___Pita

___Beer   ___Gin   ___Tequila

___Wine   ___Seltzer Water   ___Vodka

___Diet Soda   ___Soda   ___Whiskey

___Coffee / Tea   ___Energy Drink   ___Juice

___Turkey   ___Banana   ___Chinese Food

___Mexican Food   ___Fast Food   ___Salad

When you reflect on your diet, you may find that you are eating a lot less protein than you thought. This is common among my patients. Many people I see get most of their protein from milk and cheese. They also often rely on fast

food or deli meat rather than fresh, unprocessed animal meat. We live in a convenience-driven world—often moving from one obligation to the next. It is easy to rely on carbohydrate-heavy convenience foods rather than protein rich options if we allow ourselves to do it.

For those of you on strong pain killers like opiate medications, you may find that you have developed a particularly strong sweet tooth—this is common. Patients on opioids commonly gain weight and develop a preference for sweet foods. I have seen multiple patients who were placed on opiate medications by their doctor only to find relentless weight gain due to food cravings. When the opiates are weaned down and ultimately off, it is amazing how quickly their weight returns to their initial weight before the injury or illness that created their pain. They especially notice changes in their body composition, with decreased fat percentage and increased muscle mass.

In addition, the constant condition of pain stresses the body, which creates changes in the stress chemicals of your body, which not only creates an imbalance in your sugar and insulin levels but also raises the level of the stress hormone cortisol in your body. This creates a cycle of over eating and poor blood sugar control. When your blood sugar is unstable your body will experience severe cravings that only make the problem worse.

What Should I Eat?

Your goal is to eat a diet rich in healthy proteins, healthy fat, and balanced whole-food carbohydrates.

Here is a meal plan template that can help you plan your meals.

Meal Plan Template	Example
Breakfast: High Quality Protein Whole-Food Carbohydrate or Fruit Healthy Green Vegetables	Breakfast: 2 Eggs scrambled with a handful of spinach 1 cup Berries
Snack High Quality Protein	Snack 10 Almonds
Lunch High Quality Protein Whole-Food Carbohydrate Healthy Green Vegetables or Salad	Lunch 4-6 ounces of All Natural Deli Meat (Such as Boars Head "Simplicity" 2 slices Whole-Wheat Bread Sliced Cucumber
Snack High Quality Protein Whole Food Carbohydrate	Snack 1/2 cup Plain Yogurt 1/2 cup Blueberries Drizzle of Honey if the Yogurt is too tart for you
Dinner High Quality Protein Vegetables Salad	Dinner 4-6 ounces Grilled Chicken 1/2 to 1 cup Roasted Broccoli Salad dressed with home-made olive oil and balsamic vinegar

As much as possible, you want to eliminate processed food and sugars from your diet. Processed foods are usually heavy in carbohydrates and loaded with preservatives and fillers. You will find that fresh, healthy food will fill you up faster and keep you satisfied longer. These foods will also have the greatest influence on decreasing inflammation.

Know Your Protein!

The ideal protein sources will come directly from the healthiest animals you can find. Why? Because if your animal is fat, inflamed, and sick and on antibiotics or pumped full of hormones and generally unhealthy from the food that it ate, it will have an inflammatory effect on your body as well. Look for organic, free-range, wild, or grass-fed options. Salmon is a particular pain-fighting powerhouse because it is loaded with anti-inflammatory omega-3 fatty acids.

In bygone times (and even today in idyllic locations), people would buy their cows and hens from farmers they knew. Today, healthy protein sources are widely available—even budget friendly stores like Aldi have options for the health-conscious shopper. There's no need to break the bank at specialty stores. If you can't find these options in your area, then focus on getting the highest-quality protein you can—for example eat grilled chicken breasts and fresh or freshly frozen fish you cook and season yourself rather than processed deli meats, hamburgers, hot dogs, or precooked frozen fish that you find in the freezer aisle.

Pain-Pausing Produce!

I was recently driving through rural Missouri during the peak of summer. We stopped to get some snacks at a community grocery store. Despite being surrounded by productive farms, I was shocked at the shortage of fresh fruits and vegetables. The stamp "Grown in Mexico" boldly caught my eye as I scanned the strawberries (even though it was June and peak strawberry season for the region). The best produce is fresh produce that is in-season and grown organically, and as close to your home as possible. Some regions of the country have a food desert—meaning that, like the grocery store I encountered in a rural area of Missouri, the local distributors cannot effectively supply fresh, whole food. If this is your situation, then I encourage you to find solutions. If you are in a metropolitan area and you cannot find fresh produce, drive a little farther to an area that is better served. If you are from a more rural area, then find a source for fruits and vegetables to supplement what you can obtain at the grocery store. Look for farmers markets or consider participating in a farm share or CSA. You can even grow some yourself, depending on the season and your region.

Produce in the form of fruits and vegetables is loaded with antioxidants and vitamins that can improve your health. Look for items that have diverse, deep colors and are at the peak of ripeness.

Some particularly anti-inflammatory produce:

| Almonds | Cauliflower | Spinach |
| Avocados | Garlic | Strawberries |

Blueberries	Ginger	Sweet Potatoes
Brazil Nuts	Hot Pepper	Thyme
Broccoli	Red Grapes	Walnuts
Brussels Sprouts		

Considerations for Carbohydrates

Over the past ten years, carbohydrates have gotten quite the bum rap. When you are trying to eat to end inflammation, you absolutely need to be mindful of the sources of sugar in your diet. Sugar will create inflammation. However, don't unnecessarily eliminate all carbohydrates from your diet.

Focus on eating whole grain sources of complex carbohydrates. The most common of these are whole wheat, steel-cut oats, and brown rice. You can also experiment with more exotic grains like quinoa, barley, millet, or amaranth. In place of grains, you can substitute anti-oxidant rich fruits that are carbohydrate rich and starchy vegetables like sweet potatoes.

Be careful of portions. It is easy to overdo it with carbohydrates!

Change Your Eating habits, Change Your Life

Choosing a healthy diet is one of the most effective measures you can make to decrease your chances for diseases such as heart disease and cancer. Now you have learned the impact these lifestyle changes can have on your pain and the chronic inflammation in your diet, you have one more reason to make changes that serve you. Eating a nutritious and healthy diet is just one more way that you can show up for yourself and regain the confidence that you can conquer your pain!

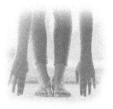

Chapter 6

Nourish Your Mind

Increasingly in the media you may have heard about the new trend toward mindfulness and meditation. This isn't simply some wellness fad or new age gimmick—meditation and mindfulness have their roots in many ancient cultures and religions. Research projects about the health benefits of mindfulness practice have exploded in the past ten years, bringing the concepts of mindfulness and meditation center stage in terms of their possibilities to improve human suffering. The process of becoming more mindful in your daily life is associated with marked decreases in stress hormones and can decrease the intensity of your pain experience.

There have also been several research studies that have demonstrated that mindfulness practices and meditation actually improve depression symptoms as well as quality of life.

What an amazing feature of our amazing minds! Our minds and our bodies are intimately connected, and the regular practice of mindfulness and meditation will decrease your anxiety, tendency toward depression, and pain-related drug utilization.

A mindfulness and meditation practice can be undertaken in just a small amount of time during the day. It is best, however, to practice on a regular basis because you do need to grow accustomed to the techniques for maximum benefit.

Mindfulness and meditation don't have to take over your whole life. I recommend working toward twenty minutes per day. However, start small, try to practice one of the exercises for five minutes per day at first. Build up to twenty minutes. Again, the most important part is to practice on a regular basis and in a way that's meaningful and comfortable to you. Build this into your routine, put it on your calendar, and show up!

Mindfulness or Meditation: What's the Difference?

The terms *mindfulness* and *meditation* are often used interchangeably. The debate about the differences between them could be the subject of its own book, and I am uncertain about its relevance here. Mindfulness can be a formal practice or an informal lifestyle. Informal practice of mindfulness involves being more aware of everything around you. It is something you do throughout the day, without specifically setting aside time for it. Informal mindfulness is a powerful tool to engage on a regular basis.

Formal practice of mindfulness refers to a type of meditation where one sets aside time with the purpose of being aware of what is happening in the present. It involves acceptance of the body and its surroundings. It involves the appreciation of the world around us. It involves living in the moment rather than waiting for the next update on our newsfeed.

For the purposes of this book, I use the terms *mindfulness* and *meditation* interchangeably. I want to introduce you to these practices and help you implement them in your lives.

I will introduce you to several beginning mindfulness meditations to get you started in your regular practice.

Mindful Breathing

Sit in a quiet place in the most comfortable position that you can find. Your eyes can be open or closed. Set a timer on your phone for your intended timeframe; start with five to seven minutes. Take a few deep breaths and feel your chest expanding and the air filling your lungs. Focus on that feeling. Then exhale and feel the air leaving your lungs as your chest drops. You do not need to adjust your breath, just be aware of the breath as it enters and leaves your body. As you continue breathing you may notice that your mind begins to wander. This is normal. As thoughts enter your mind, gently redirect your thoughts back to your breath. Sometimes saying a word to yourself like "breathing" or "thinking" is helpful for the redirection.

Don't be too hard on yourself if you have a lot of difficulty redirecting your wandering mind. That is precisely why you need these exercises! It will become easier, and with regular practice, you will actually create new, healthy, pathways in your brain!

The Body Awareness Scan

This practice builds on the breath exercise and creates greater awareness of your body. I would approach this exercise when you are comfortable doing the breathing exercise for at least ten minutes.

Start by taking a few mindful breaths as described in the last exercise. After you have effectively turned your attention to your breathing, start focusing on your body from head to toe. Evaluate each body part systematically.

Start with your head; how does your head feel? Do you have pain or tension in your head? If you have tension, try to release it. If you have pain, then focus on it for a moment with curiosity. How does it feel? Is it throbbing, nagging, or something else? Take a moment and accept it. We aren't here to fix or change anything. We are only here to gain awareness.

- Move to your neck. How does your neck feel?
- Your shoulders and arms.
- Focus on your whole upper body for a moment.
- Then move your awareness to your mid-back, your chest, and then to your stomach, then to your low back.
- and your buttocks,
- Then take a moment to consider your whole torso. How does it feel?
- Move on to your legs and allow yourself to become aware of them. Do they ache, twitch, cramp?
- How do your hips feel? Your knees, your ankles, your toes?
- Spend a few more moments observing your whole body breathing in and out as one.
- Open your eyes if they were closed.
- How do you feel?

You can modify this body scan. You can limit to one body part of interest—for example if you notice pain in your shoulder you can perform this exercise on only your shoulder. Likewise, you can do this exercise and pay attention to specific body parts that are not in pain.

Pain Acceptance Meditation

This meditation is best used in the moments when you're experiencing your worst pain: an eight to ten out of ten on your pain scale. You can begin in the same way as the first exercise sitting quietly and comfortably and focusing on your breathing.

Start by finding a comfortable position in a quiet place. Close your eyes. Focus your attention to your breathing and the sensation of the breath entering and leaving your body. After doing this for five to ten breaths, focus down on the area of your body that is causing you the most pain.

How does the pain feel?

Be curious about your pain as you as you allow your mind to focus on it. Get to know it. How does the pain feel? Is it throbbing, constant, burning sharp, poking, or how can you describe it? Does your pain restrict your movement? Is your pain in just one body part or is it affecting multiple parts? Systematically direct your attention to each body part affected. Don't try to interfere with the pain or try to analyze it; just get to know it and accept it.

Throw Away Your Triggers

This is another exercise for when you experience severe pain between an eight and a ten. Start again by finding a comfortable position and centering on your breath. Examine your pain. What emotion are you feeling right now? What were you doing immediately before the pain started? Were you having a strong emotion? Were you angry or frustrated? Were you challenging your body to try something new? I want you to think about what triggered your pain, and I want you to imagine seeing the scene play out on a screen. I want you to imagine throwing the screen away. Now with a new screen, imagine the same scene. This time, however, you complete the task without pain. You are successful. What emotions do you feel? Lean into how you feel conquering the task. Lean into the visualization of you achieving your goal.

Recenter your breathing and redirect back to your body. Has your pain changed? If your pain is still severe, I want you to imagine an empty vessel with a strong captain steering the boat. I want you to visualize taking the pain from your body and placing it in the vessel. I want you to imagine your pain leaving your body and filling the vessel, and the vessel simply disappearing in the horizon, directed away by the ship captain.

For my Christian readers, this visualization is particularly effective when you visualize the outstretched hands of Jesus. Imagine putting all your physical pain in Jesus's hands and imagine him lovingly taking it from you.

Mindful Moments

As you become more mindful with regular practice of these exercises, you may find opportunities to build mindfulness into your daily life. The important thing is mindfulness is most effective when it is the acceptance of what is. Visualization of what you want your present to be is also effective. However, don't dwell on the past or relive what could have been done differently. Don't invest energy in dissecting what you could have said or how you could have felt in a given moment. Instead, welcome and accept whatever thoughts and feelings you have in the moment.

For example, if you experienced severe pain when you try to do something new that you feel should be within your reasonable physical capacity to achieve—like, for instance, throwing a baseball with your child—reflect for a moment with curiosity on what pain limited you. If you want to perform a visualization, visualize yourself easily and painlessly performing the activity you wish.

No Experience Necessary

One of the remarkable things about mindfulness meditation and its application to pain management is that research participants have shown improvements even when the have had no experience with these techniques before the study. It really doesn't take much time to get comfortable with practicing meditation once you start doing it regularly.

Additionally, there are some studies that suggest that these practices have more power than meditation. In a recent study looking at participants who practice meditation regularly for a period of twenty minutes at a time, three times per week, they have demonstrated predictable decrease in pain perceptions by greater than 20 percent, regardless of the medications that they take.

Studies have also compared participants administered either a placebo saline solution or a strong powerful painkiller called the naloxone. These participants were invited into four groups: (a) meditation plus naloxone, (b) no meditation plus naloxone, (c) meditation plus saline, and (d) control plus saline.

The findings in the group are remarkable. Those participants who participated in meditation and took medication demonstrated reduced pain ratings by 24 percent; those patients who practiced meditation plus were administered saline reduced their pain scores by 21 percent. In comparison, *both* the medication and saline groups without meditation reported increases of pain. All groups who meditated had measurable decreases in reported pain score, but even the patients taking strong medication reported that their pain increased compared to the meditating groups receiving saline! This suggests that there are unique brain pathways that mediate pain signals that occur with meditation.

Mindfulness will not eliminate the structural pain that you may experience. However, even if your condition requires surgical intervention, the focus on both breathing and relaxation as well as awareness of your body and acceptance of the present moment decrease your stress hormones in reaction to your injury and increase your endorphins (feel-good hormones). This process decreases your need for strong medications and may increase your likelihood of a positive outcome from surgery.

Perhaps the most compelling reason for you to start these exercises today is that there are no side effects. The only risk is the loss of time you invest. All evidence points that you will reclaim that lost time by spending more time free from suffering. Why not try it today?

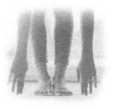

Chapter 7

Exercise Freely

It is common in my practice that I encounter people who, after an injury or after experiencing long-term pain, fear movement. Their bodies have revolted against them for so long, and sometimes the slightest engagement in activity is met with severe and unrelenting pain. I find that I can help patients face this fear of movement in similar ways to other challenges we've talked about in other chapters.

A lot of times, I find that people have unrealistic expectations of themselves after periods of deconditioning. They expect too much from themselves, too soon. Their desire for movement often doesn't match their physical limitations upon their initial reintroduction to exercise and they "overdo it," setting themselves back further.

I find that exercise in these cases is best managed with small, simple and achievable goals. I think it is important to celebrate your accomplishments, no matter how small, as they occur.

This chapter will address realistic expectations and give you an overview of some core movements to implement to help and encourage your body to function and move with more efficiency.

There are three components to this plan: (1) stretching, (2) strengthening, and (3) aerobic conditioning. I encourage you to discuss these exercises with your doctor or physical therapist to make sure that they are appropriate for your specific condition.

Stretching

Strength and flexibility are closely connected. When recovering after a period of inactivity due to pain or injury, it's very important to maintain flexibility in your muscles. Below is a series of stretches that may help you. These stretches are targeted for back and neck pain, because that's what I see most commonly in my practice. There are many other exercises for other body areas that may benefit you. You can talk to your doctor or physical therapist about some stretches that might serve you based on your physical conditioning, pain, and injury. The following exercises may be helpful for your body, regardless of where you've been injured, as the back and neck support our entire body. If you would like video or images of these exercises, they are all common and easily accessible if you search on the internet.

1. Neck Stretch
Move your head gently to the left and then the right, hold each position for two to five seconds, breathing deeply throughout the motions.

Then gently move your head to look up and down, using care not to tilt your head too far backward, again hold each position for two to five seconds.

Repeat each position three times.

2. Cat and Camel
Lower yourself to the floor, on a thick carpet or mat, and support your body on your hands and knees. Slowly stretch your spine up toward the ceiling, like the arched back of an angry cat. Feel the stretch in your lower back, hold for ten to twenty seconds.

Then, lower your midsection down, like the valley between two camel humps. Hold this position for ten seconds. Then repeat, five to ten times, building toward fifteen repetitions.

3. Legs to Chest Stretch

Lie on your back and bring your left knee to your chest, hold for ten to twenty seconds.

Repeat with your right leg.

Repeat with both legs.

Strengthening

Your core strength is imperative to your maintenance of proper posture. Posture can influence multiple painful conditions. Below are a series of exercises that will help you strengthen some of the small core muscles of your back and neck and help restore your posture so that the burden on your bones, ligaments and discs in your back is diminished.

1. Chin Tuck Retraction

Stand with your shoulders back and slowly draw your chin back so that your ears line up with your shoulders. Your forehead should not tilt up or down with this movement.

2. Bird Dog

Lower yourself to the floor (on a mat or carpet) onto your hands and knees. Tighten your abdominal muscles with your neck looking to the floor and your back in a neutral position. Slowly extend your left leg behind you while extending your right arm in front of you. Don't let your back arch! Hold this position for five seconds. Lower your leg and arm back to the ground. Repeat with the opposite side.

If you cannot stay balanced and extend your leg/arm without arching your back, then just lift your knee and hand a few inches off the ground and work up to fully extending the arm and leg. Repeat five to ten times.

3. Dead Bug

Lie on your back with your hips and knees bent to a ninety-degree angle and your calves parallel to the floor. Elevate your arms to a ninety-degree angle with your torso. Take a deep breath in, and exhale, pulling your spine toward the floor into a neutral position and contract your abdominal muscles. Keeping your abdominal muscles tight and your heels flexed, slowly extend your right arm over your head, and straighten your left leg away from you until your heel touches the floor. Return to the starting position and repeat with the opposite arm and leg. Repeat this exercise for a total of five to ten times per side.

If you don't feel strong enough or coordinated enough to work both your arms and legs at the same time, try this exercise first moving just your legs and work toward moving both your arms and your legs.

4. Hip Bridge

Lie on your back with your knees bent, and your feet flat on the floor shoulder width apart. Place your arms at your sides. Take a deep breath in and tighten your abdominal muscles while exhaling. Press your heels into the ground, squeeze the muscles in your buttocks, and lift your hips off the floor. Try to make one diagonal line from your shoulders to your knees. Hold for one to three seconds; then lower your buttocks back to the ground. This exercise is most effective when you move slowly. Repeat ten to fifteen times.

Aerobic Conditioning

When embarking on an exercise program after a period of inactivity due to pain, I recommend starting with small, reasonable and achievable goals rather than trying to resume activities you once were able to do easily. When you push yourself too hard, not only will you risk worsened pain, but you also risk becoming sad, frustrated, or disappointed in your body for not doing the things that it used to be able to do. Celebrate small accomplishments on a daily basis for the best results!

My recommendation is to work toward thirty minutes of aerobic conditioning in the form of walking, swimming, dancing, water aerobics, or other activities that increase your heart rate as your body allows. If walking in your neighborhood or on a treadmill is too strenuous given your physical condition, then I recommend walking in a lazy river or in four feet of water in a pool. This will essentially remove the force of a significant portion of your weight on your muscles and joints. If you're particularly lucky, the fitness center or a physical therapist in your neighborhood may have a zero-gravity treadmill or a treadmill placed in a pool that can help recondition your body by slowly and intentionally adjusting the amount of your body weight you must carry during activity.

The easiest way to start reconditioning is with walking in your neighborhood or gently dancing and moving to enjoyable music. Depending on how long it has been since you've engaged in regular activity, choose a starting point that is reasonable and achievable for you. This may be five minutes, or it may be twenty. Perhaps you're able to move for thirty minutes without experiencing increased pain already, but you just haven't done so regularly.

First, you need to schedule your times of exercise. This is time that you have to save for yourself. Make a plan and show up for yourself. Put it on your calendar.

Second, I recommend setting a timer for your initial goal of movement. Choose a time that is no more than half of the amount of time that you feel that you may be able to move continuously without increasing your pain afterward. For instance, if you feel that you are likely able to move regularly for ten minutes, then start by setting a timer for five minutes. I suggest making your goal as achievable as possible, because creating a pattern of exercising regularly is more important than the time you invest. You will build up your time as your body allows. Just show up for yourself to exercise regularly. Celebrate yourself each time you show up! Way to go! You are moving!

Now, go outside or get on a treadmill, find a lazy river at the local pool, or pick out your favorite song and move for your targeted amount of time each day. When you know you are comfortable with the time that you are moving, and you are not experiencing severe increases in pain that last for days after your movement, increase your goal movement time by two minutes.

Be patient with yourself! Perhaps when you start, you can only move for two or three minutes without experiencing an increase in your symptoms. That's OK! You have to start somewhere! You are moving more than you did yesterday. With scheduled, gradual, and reasonable increases in your activity level and working toward a goal of thirty minutes of movement three to five times per week, you will begin to trust your body with movement again. You will feel better as you consistently work toward small activity goals. You will be able to make significant gains in your physical abilities without increasing your pain.

If these exercises are still too strenuous for you, consider learning tai chi. Tai chi is a form of movement that focuses on fluid motions with minimal impact on your body. People of all ages and body sizes can participate in tai chi with relatively little difficulty, and it is appropriate for all levels of fitness and even those who are paralyzed, disabled, or relegated to a wheelchair can achieve benefits from tai chi.

Given the unique movements that may be new to you, I recommend teaming up with an instructor in tai chi for at least the beginning of your learning process and practice. After you've done several sessions and feel confident performing the movements on your own a video or at home practice may suffice. Certainly, if no instructor is available in your area, then there are free videos available online, and also DVDs available for purchase. Regardless of which activity you choose, and your level of fitness starting out, I find the most important part of an exercise program for patients with chronic pain is celebrating accomplishments and setting goals. Think about a marathon runner training for a marathon. When she first starts, she may be able to run only one mile continuously. But with strategically planned increases in running distances, and regular and consistent practice, she is able to achieve the unimaginable twenty-six miles of constant running. This ability isn't formed in one day of training, and this level of athleticism is not achieved without some expense of pain.

When you can focus your mindset on celebrating the small achievements that you may be able to create with their body, you will be able to work toward amazing goals. While you may never have a goal to run a marathon, making a goal and creating a regular, strategic, and reasonable schedule to achieve it—and celebrating each step you are able to achieve during the process—will create amazing results and minimize your pain with movement.

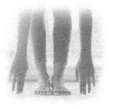

Chapter 8

Work Matters

When you develop pain that started due to an injury or accident that occurred at work, inevitably, the question "When will I return to work?" or "Will I ever return to work?" comes up. The pursuit of your career, trade, or profession creates a significant amount of positive health effects. Your physical and mental health are both generally improved through regular work. It's to be expected that you want to get back to work as soon as possible. Any work, whether paid or voluntary, helps you maintain your confidence and self-esteem. Additionally, work rewards you financially. Work helps you maintain a consistent routine. Your job allows you to interact with other people and builds a support system with other people.

Work gives you a sense of pride, identity, and personal achievement. In general, people who are working tend to enjoy healthier and happier lives than those who are not working.

One of my favorite quotes was written by Max Ehrmann in his Poem "Desiderata"—"Keep interested in your career, however humble; it is a real possession in the changing fortunes of time." Indeed, your career is your possession. You have invested your time in developing your skills and education in your chosen field. It is disappointing to face potential disability that would prevent you from applying your skills to your profession!

However, sometimes employers let their employees down. What if you feel like your employer hasn't been supportive to you since you were injured? What if you have fears about returning to work?

Perhaps you are afraid of getting laid off or fired upon your return. Perhaps you are afraid of reinjury. Perhaps you are afraid of some retribution from your coworkers.

Try to set those fears aside. It's important to follow your doctor's recommendations in terms of the activities you can perform upon your return. Advocate for yourself and know your restrictions. Often, employees may be asked to extend themselves outside of their restrictions

because their supervisor simply doesn't remember what specific restrictions the employee has. Sometimes, the employee might interpret this as purposeful interference in their recovery. Recognize this as a negative thought you are having. It is far more likely that your employer is excited to have you back at work, thrilled you are doing well and is happy to help you prevent reinjury by honoring your restrictions.

It is easy to lean into negative thoughts that help to create your fears with regard to your return to work. One of the negative impacts of pain that becomes chronic is the development of fears and negative thoughts regarding one's ability to return to work. This occurs regardless of whether your pain initiate from an injury at work or at home.

Your negative thoughts may lure you to the idea of pursuing disability. Certainly, there are some injuries that result in life-changing disability. I have seen patients with even the most devastating of injuries return successfully to work. I have seen patients who have had unbelievable injuries return to work. The overall benefits of work outweigh significantly the financial impact that any disability benefit could provide. You are financially, physically, and emotionally better off working and advancing your skills than not.

When people suffer from periods of unemployment, such as that during the recovery from an injury. Significan mental health improvements occur as soon as they retu to work. Studies on patients who have sought disabi

for their painful conditions show higher rates of anxiety, depression, and divorce within three years of initiating disability benefits. Disability puts strain on relationships and worsens the negative thoughts and emotions in the person who is disabled as well as his or her spouse.

However humble your education or however meager your financial reward is from your work, realize that the investment of time in your work duties is an investment in yourself.

There are times where your current job may not be able to modify your duties to meet your restrictions. In these cases, it can be hard to see a path forward. What will you do? What will happen to you?

Consider occupational counseling. Sometimes an experienced occupational counselor can give you some good options of potential new careers you could pursue. It is amazing the diverse tasks that humans perform in exchange for money. Regardless of education level, there may be forms of employment that do not require the same physical demands as your current job.

Sometimes there is no other option than to pursue disability to secure you and your family's financial solvency. If disability is the only option, then I urge you to find some volunteer opportunity. There are endless opportunities. For example, you could talk to your doctor about becoming a patient resource for others who are suffering from your similar condition or injury. Anything that allows you to

develop a routine and interact with others can provide you with benefits.

When you return to work, pay attention to your thoughts and be realistic about any limitations that your body may have in your recovery. It is easy to become frustrated with yourself when you cannot perform with the same efficiency as you did prior to your accident. Strive for improvement but be gentle with yourself. Rather than feeling negatively about yourself and your body not being able to do the things that you used to do, rejoice and celebrate the things that you are able to do.

Celebrate your achievements that come from meeting small professional goals. As an employed individual, you will enjoy improved mental health, take less medication, and (as shown by some studies) have a longer life expectancy than those who remain unemployed.

I don't have to tell you the many financial benefits of work. Continuing your work allows you to have the financial freedom to explore your interests outside of work. What do you love to do in your free time? A return to work will make your hobbies and interests more accessible to you.

What gives you joy out of your work? Is it the interpersonal interactions with your coworkers? Is it the challenge that your employment affords you? Is it your pride in the fact that you're "the best at what you do"?

As part of your thought reflection practice, consider your thoughts regarding work.

Were you injured at work? Do you feel that somehow your employer failed you? Do you feel that somehow your medical treatment was flawed while recovering from your injury?

Consider all these negative thoughts and their impact that they are having on your physical recovery. Consider that these thoughts could be creating a false sense of reality. The reality is the contributions that you make to your employer matter. It is unlikely that there is any intentional external force that is limiting your recovery.

As you continue to examine your thoughts, focus further on the culture at work. How did you like your job before? Was your work a positive environment? Was it a stressful and pressured environment? If the answer is the latter, then I would encourage you to reflect on what strategies you could try to shift the culture to a more positive environment. You could look at this as an opportunity to change gears and find employment that makes you feel valued, secure, supported, and respected.

There are many work cultures that create a positive, thriving, and healthy environment. With your motivation and determination, you can return to work and thrive.

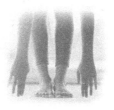

Chapter 9

Supplements for Success

I'm frequently asked about the multiple nutritional supplements on the market that claim to help improve pain. The following is a summary of some of the most commonly available and frequently requested supplements that I feel can create the biggest improvement to your pain. This is by no means an exhaustive list. There are many other supplements on the market that claim to improve pain. I encourage you to work with your doctor and discuss these options as well as others to see if they may work within an individualized treatment protocol for you.

Omega-3 Fatty Acids

Omega-3 fatty acids are powerfully anti-inflammatory and can help improve multiple conditions in the human body. They are a "good fat" and are prevalent in walnuts, other tree nuts, flaxseeds, chia seeds, and cold-water fish as well as over-the-counter supplements.

Omega-3 fatty acids have an incredible impact on human health. They add fuel for both our bodies and our brains. They can fight depression and anxiety and improve your overall health. They can promote brain development during pregnancy. They decrease the risk of development of autism, ADHD, and cerebral palsy. They improve the risk factors for heart disease and strokes. They can reduce the symptoms of ADHD in children. They can reduce the symptoms of metabolic syndrome, and most importantly to me, they fight inflammation

As we previously addressed, inflammation is incredibly important in the mediation of pain. Inflammation contributes to not only almost every chronic Western disease, including cancer and heart disease, but also is integral to the production of chemicals that mediate pain.

Omega-3 fatty acids can be prescribed by your doctor or can be obtained from your pharmacy. For pain management, I recommend a fish oil supplement that is high in eicosapentaenoic acid (EPA). The best way to get your omega-3 fatty acids is by eating wild-caught fatty fish, such as salmon, at least two times per week. Supplementation is important also, as it is difficult to consume enough salmon to have therapeutic effect on pain. There are a variety of prescription-strength fish oil pills marketed under different brand names. These medications are prescribed to control triglyceride levels in people with elevated cholesterol, which has positive impacts on cardiovascular health. They tend to be expensive and may not be covered by your insurance. Many of the brand-name options are relatively high in EPA and may result in greater decrease of the inflammation in your body. The general goal is at least two grams of omega-3 fatty acids per day. Over the counter supplements are acceptable and more cost-effective, although may have to take more capsules to achieve the necessary dose. The FDA recommends that omega-3 fatty acid supplements be limited to no more than three grams per day

Be careful with fish oil, because it can thin your blood, so if you're about to engage in a surgical intervention or injection, it's best to avoid omega-3 fatty acid supplements for the week prior to these procedures.

Probiotics

Probiotics are the good bacteria that live in your gut. Poor gut health can play a role in contributing to multiple health conditions, including ADHD, autism, and unexplained weight gain. The bacteria in your guy is integral to your immune system. Multiple factors can create negative effects to our gut bacteria. High carbohydrate diets, eating a limited mixture of fruits and vegetables, drinking too much alcohol, a sedentary lifestyle, cigarette smoking, stress, poor sleep, and frequent use of hand sanitizers and antibiotics all create a negative effect on the balance of good and bad bacteria in your gut. Implementing any of these measures can create positive impact.

Probiotics—the good bacteria we need to populate our gut—are live microorganisms that can provide potent health benefits when are when they are consumed. Having a healthy gut bacteria balance (a healthy microbiome) reduces inflammation, eases anxiety and depression, improves acne and rosacea, and strengthens your immune system (among other good things). The benefits don't just stop there. People who take probiotics regularly and eliminate the things that harm the good bacteria will have improvements in digestive functioning and athletic performance by increasing the absorption of positive nutrients so that muscles can function appropriately. A healthy microbiome can prevent wrinkles and aging, too. Bonus!

It may take up to twelve weeks of regular use of probiotic supplements to start to see the health benefits. Within thirty days, you might start to see subtle changes. Take a probiotic supplement on an empty stomach in the morning. There are many commercially available over-the-counter bacterial supplements. You want to start with a supplement that has at least thirty billion colony-forming units, or CFUs. Look for bacterial species such as

Bifidobacterium and *Lactobacillus* GG. The more species, the better; some supplements have as many as twelve or more different strains of good bacteria.

Probiotics are usually tolerated well by patients. However, you may have a few negative effects when you start. You can have a temporary increase of gas, bloating, constipation, or thirst. Some supplements may have additives that can trigger food intolerances or allergies, and not every bacterial strain works for all patients. If you fail to respond to a given supplement, try another brand with a different mix of bacterial species.

Vitamin D

Most inhabitants of the United States are deficient in vitamin D. Vitamin D is usually produced by our skin in response to being exposed to sunlight. Because of this, darker skinned individuals and fair skinned individuals who frequently use high-SPF sunscreen are particularly susceptible. Americans are pretty much guaranteed to be deficient unless they frequently avoid sunscreen and actively spend a lot of time outdoors with sleeveless clothing. Vitamin D also occurs naturally in a few foods, including some fish, fish oils, and egg yolks. It is also usually supplemented in our milk. Vitamin D helps the body use calcium from the diet.

Historically, vitamin D deficiency was associated with rickets, which is a disease where the bone tissue isn't properly mineralized. This causes soft bones and skeletal deformities.

Vitamin D has been found to protect against a whole array of health problems—fibromyalgia and chronic pain, in particular. Vitamin D deficiency can also impact your risk of cardiovascular disease, cognitive impairment, asthma, and cancer. Patients with proper diet vitamin D levels have improvement in their control of type 2 diabetes, hypertension, insulin resistance, and multiple sclerosis.

Vitamin D is best supplemented in the form of vitamin D3. If you do not know your vitamin D level, ask your doctor to check it for you. I recommend a starting point of one thousand international units (IU) per day until you know your level. In general, patients with vitamin D deficiency need five thousand IU per day to correct vitamin D deficiency. Some people with severely low levels or difficulty remembering to take their pills may benefit from higher weekly doses of fifty thousand IU per week. Your goal is to get your levels greater than 30 ng/mL, and preferably greater than 40 ng/mL.

Calcium and Magnesium

Magnesium functions as a muscle relaxant. Due to this function, magnesium is known to reduce pain by relaxing muscles and decreasing spasms. Magnesium eases the pain of tense muscles. Magnesium deficiency can create chronic inflammation and supplementing with magnesium can create significant improvements in nerve pain. It has the biggest impact on pain related to fibromyalgia, as well as

Lyme disease and lupus, and decreases muscle cramps that are especially common at night. Magnesium deficiency is associated with weakness in the joints and abnormalities in cartilage as well osteoporosis and rheumatoid arthritis.

Magnesium is best absorbed through the skin. I recommend use of a topical magnesium oil to be applied to the "hot spots" of your body, including the backs of your knees and inside of your elbows at night. Use of Epsom salts in your bath can also increase the magnesium absorption through the skin.

You can supplement magnesium orally as well. I recommend a supplement called Natural Calm that you take at night according to the package directions. Natural Calm can have the added benefit of helping you fall asleep at night. It is widely available at your local pharmacy.

If you take an oral tablet of magnesium, always look for one in a 2:1 ratio of calcium to magnesium. Magnesium can loosen stools and is often used as a laxative (think of milk of magnesia). This effects its absorption through your gut. Calcium has a mild constipating effect.

Calcium and magnesium supplements are commercially available at your local pharmacy.

B Vitamins

B vitamins are essential for nerve health and supplementation creates improvements in a variety of nerve-related conditions. B vitamins are also nutritionally important and they help manufacturer red blood cells.

The vitamins B1, B6, and B12 seem to have the greatest impact for neuropathic pain. You can obtain these vitamins from the foods you eat as well as supplementation.

Vitamin B1

Vitamin B1 is particularly high in foods such as whole grains, dairy products, and red meat. It is also synthesized by healthy gut bacteria. Thiamine (Vitamin B1) is converted to its active form where it functions as an enzyme for carbohydrate metabolism in the brain. This makes it a key player in energy metabolism and the processing of glucose.

Vitamin B12

Vitamin B12 is also synthesized in some gut bacteria and is found in animal products such as fish, beef, poultry, and dairy products. Vitamin B12 is required in the body for multiple processes within the body, including cell reproduction, cell growth, and the creation of blood cells. This feature explains why B12 deficiency can be associated with anemia.

Vitamin B6

Vitamin B6 deficiency is less common than deficiencies of B1 and B12. It is most common in alcoholics, smokers, obese people, and people who suffer from liver and kidney problems. Vitamin B6 has both anti-inflammatory and antioxidant properties. Adequate vitamin B6 also influences your mood.

How to Take Your B Vitamins

B vitamins are water-soluble vitamins so it's hard to overdose on them. Find a B complex with at least Vitamin B1, B6, and B12. Some people do not absorb vitamin B12 orally. If you don't see effects from supplementation, consider a spray or lozenge you can place under the tongue (sublingual).

Melatonin

Melatonin is actually a hormone, not a vitamin. Melatonin is the hormone that we produce in our bodies when we prepare for sleep. There is some suggestion that melatonin not only can create improvement in sleep disturbances caused by pain but also has some impact on the neuropathic pain itself. Melatonin can decrease the sleep disturbances created by jetlag while traveling and can correct sleep patterns that are disrupted due to shift work.

Melatonin supplements appear to be safe when you use them short term. However, you want to be cautious if you're using these medications for more than a month or two. If you find that you are using this supplement for chronic insomnia, you should consider discussing with your doctor a sleep study to confirm the cause of your insomnia.

Melatonin has the biggest effect at reducing the time it takes to fall asleep rather than truly keeping you asleep. You want to try to take it roughly thirty minutes before going to bed.

Doses between 0.5 mg and 5 mg seem to work. Start with the lowest dose you can find, then work up gradually to 3 to 5 mg. The benefits are not typically dose dependent, so taking more than 5 mg will not help you fall asleep faster.

Valerian Root

Valerian root can be brewed into a tincture or tea, and it creates a sedative effect that helps relax you and can improve your sleep quality. It is a safe and effective sleep aid that can reduce the time that it takes to fall asleep and help you sleep better.

Valerian root seems to be most effective when you take it regularly at the same time for two or more weeks.

Keep in mind that in the United States, herbal supplements are not monitored by the Food and Drug Administration the same way medications are, so you want to be certain that you get your valerian root from a high-quality manufacturer.

Chronic use of valerian root has the added benefit of decreasing your blood pressure and improving anxiety.

You can buy an organic valerian root tea supplement at your local supermarket, or you can take the supplement in the form of a pill. Follow the package directions for the product you choose.

Boswellia

Boswellia is an herbal supplement also known as Indian frankincense. *Boswellia* has been used for centuries in Asian and African folk medicine to treat chronic inflammatory illnesses and improve pain conditions. It can reduce the inflammation from conditions like osteoarthritis, rheumatoid arthritis, asthma, and inflammatory bowel disease. It can be an effective painkiller and can also have the added benefit of preventing the loss of cartilage and destruction in the joints.

There are many studies that suggest that it is even useful in treating certain cancers such as leukemia and breast cancer. The impacts of *Boswellia* on knee pain have been researched. In one study of nearly ninety patients with known knee arthritis, 100 percent of those patients reported a decrease in knee pain after supplementing with *Boswellia* for ninety days. Participants reported an increase in the distance of walking, and aspiration from their knee revealed lower levels of the cartilage degrading enzymes. *Boswellia* also positively influences other medical conditions such as Crohn's disease, ulcerative colitis, and asthma.

Generally, I would suggest finding a product that contains at least 60 percent *Boswellia* acids and taking at least 250 mg per day. Follow the directions on the package that you choose, as availability of the active form varies between manufacturers. *Boswellia* reduces pain rapidly, often within one week of supplementation.

Avoid *Boswellia* if you're pregnant, as it may induce miscarriage. It can also stimulate the blood flow in the uterus and pelvis and therefore accelerating menstrual flow. If you're taking nonsteroidal anti-inflammatory medications, be aware that *Boswellia* can decrease the effects of these medications.

Capsaicin

Capsaicin is the active agent in hot peppers that gives them their spice. This supplement, when used by spicing up your foods or topically applied in the form of a cream, can have profound benefits and improvements in pain. Capsaicin is thought to stimulate the release of a chemical called Substance P that helps transmit pain signals from sensory nerve fibers to the brain. After you repetitively apply capsaicin, the local stores of Substance P become depleted in nerve fibers in that area. That means the nerves can't transmit as many pain signals as they did before.

Topical application does create a burning sensation. Be prepared! Remember, the burning sensation is not causing you any harm. It's not creating a rash or reaction. It's an expected side effect of this potent anti-inflammatory. The uncomfortable burning sensation should lessen within a few minutes, and it will also become less prevalent with repeated topical applications.

There are very few side effects of capsaicin, and topical capsaicin has implications to improve arthritis pain as well as neuropathic pain, such as that which occurs after experiencing shingles. There's a topical prescription medication called Qutenza (8% Capsaicin) that can help and be applied in your doctor's office topically to decrease localized nerve pain.

Using capsaicin along with other pain relievers, such as nonsteroidal anti-inflammatory medications like ibuprofen, seems to create a synergistic effect that improves the function of these medications.

Capsaicin applied topically must be applied four times per day because it provides only temporary relief at first. Apply enough over the painful area and rub it into your skin until it disappears. Be sure to wash your hands immediately so that you don't get any in your eyes, nose, or mouth. If you've ever chopped a jalapeño and then accidentally touched your face, you'll understand why; it will create a lot of burning in the eye or in an area of broken skin. You also will want to avoid using a heating pad on the area that you're treating. It might take a week of regular use before you feel the full effect. If you don't notice any effects on your pain after four weeks, stop using it.

Glucosamine and Chondroitin

Glucosamine and chondroitin have been implicated with improvements in pain from osteoarthritis. They create a cartilage sparing effect that limits joint pain. Glucosamine is a naturally occurring compound that is found in the cartilage.

Usually the supplements available on the market are harvested from shellfish or made in a laboratory. Glucosamine and chondroitin are generally safe. This supplement can be a safe and effective option for people who can't take nonsteroidal anti-inflammatory medications, such as anyone who has recently had gastric bypass surgery.

Glucosamine and chondroitin are not appropriate for patients who have or had shellfish allergies. The supplement can also interfere with your blood sugar metabolism. So you'll want to stop taking glucosamine two weeks before an elective surgery to prevent unwanted shifts in your blood sugar. If you are diabetic and your glucose control or HbA1c changes, consider discussing the value of continuing glucosamine and chondroitin with your doctor. If you're on a blood thinner, like warfarin, you want to be cautious because glucosamine/chondroitin may interfere or increase with the effects of the anticoagulant and increase your risk of bleeding.

Start by taking glucosamine and chondroitin in combination for approximately one month or for as long as one bottle of the medication lasts. If by the time you complete the bottle, you haven't noticed effects of this medication, there's no need to continue it, and you can stop it safely.

Turmeric

Turmeric is a potent anti-inflammatory. The active ingredient of turmeric is curcumin. Curcumin has been used as an herbal remedy for centuries. Turmeric is commonly used as a spice in Southeast Asian cuisine, especially in Indian and Thai food. Turmeric may have pain-reducing power equal to that of prescription medications. Turmeric also seems to create positive impact on Crohn's disease, ulcerative colitis, irritable bowel syndrome, rheumatoid arthritis, and post-operative inflammation. Turmeric also has powerful impact on decreasing blood sugar and improving diabetes and preventing Alzheimer's disease. Turmeric supports liver health in some cases as well.

You can purchase turmeric as a fresh root that you can grate into your food.

You can also combine turmeric, honey, peppercorns, ginger, cinnamon, and coconut milk and create "Golden Tea." Black pepper mixed with turmeric creates a synergistic anti-inflammatory effect.

Turmeric supplements are also available. You should look for turmeric supplements with black pepper extract or piperine. This helps improve the absorption of the turmeric to make it more effective. Oral turmeric supplements can be more effective than over the counter nonsteroidal anti-inflammatories, and they're not associated with the same side effects that may be associated with NSAIDs. Adults can take 400 to 600 mg of standardized curcuminoids three times per day. It may take up to eight weeks for you to notice the benefit from turmeric so be patient if you start this supplement.

Cannabidiol

Recently, I have been asked about Cannabidiol (CBD oil) more than any other supplement.

CBD oil is one of the many cannabinoids present in the cannabis plant. There are many potential therapeutic uses of CBD oil. Its potential to improve pain is just one of the many applications. Marijuana contains both THC and CBD, as well as other cannabinoids. THC is the compound that creates the mind altering "high" when one smokes or ingest it. CBD oil is not psychoactive, meaning that it doesn't change your state of mind. It also doesn't show up on commercialized drug tests.

CBD oil attaches to receptors in your brain and can have impacts on inflammation pain as well as movement effects. CBD oil is used as a complement to other medications for the treatment of epilepsy. There's also been some evidence that CBD oil can help people quit smoking. CBD has positive impacts on anxiety, mood, and insomnia.

A recent study in the *Journal of Experimental Medicine* found that CBD oil significantly reduced chronic inflammation and pain in mice and rats.

While, the THC in marijuana can trigger and amplify feelings of anxiousness, paranoia, and anxiety, CBD oil actually has a calming effect and can reduce anxiety-related behaviors in people with conditions like generalized anxiety disorder and post-traumatic stress disorder.

CBD oil derived from hemp is legal in all fifty states. There are some products that are derived from marijuana and the legality of these supplements varies. Some states may require a prescription.

Cissus Quadrangularis

An ancient Ayurvedic treatment that stimulates bone growth and is a rich source of vitamin C, *Cissus quadrangularis* can help improve pain from bony abnormalities. It can help fractured bones heal more quickly. It can improve pain from the spine. It can improve osteoporosis, osteoarthritis, and rheumatoid arthritis. It has both pain-relieving and anti-inflammatory effects. It can also aid post-workout recovery times in athletes and is used by endurance athletes.

It is believed that *Cissus* can also increase the body collagen creation and turnover rate. This has implications in delaying aging as our collagen breaks down in our skin and joints.

Look for *Cissus* supplements that have 750 mg of *Cissus* extract per pill. Take according to the package directions.

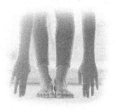

Chapter 10

What the Heck Are They Doing to Me?

When I first meet patients, they often have a lot of questions about the treatments and medications that their doctors may have ordered to help treat their conditions. I want to spend a minute just reviewing some of these for you so that you can understand some of the basis behind what we do as physicians to help treat pain.

Steroid Injections

Steroids work to diminish inflammation. If your doctor has discussed a steroid injection with you, these injections can be incredibly useful tools in the management of your pain. While the thought of having an injection might create some fear—most people, even those patients with extensive tattoos—don't like needles very much. I feel that if a steroid injection could help and control your pain symptoms and prevent you from needing surgery, that's awesome!

Surgery doesn't always alleviate pain the way we hope. In cases of anatomic problems that are creating your symptoms, there is certainly a use. However, there are usually no guarantees. No matter how excellent the surgeon (and believe me, I collaborate with some rather excellent surgeons), surgery always has its limitations.

Many patients come to me after their surgeon has suggested or ordered a steroid injection very skeptical. Why should I have the steroid injection at all? Why don't we just "fix" the problem?

Here's the thing: in most cases, the problem is actually the inflammation itself not the structural problems that your doctor may have found on an MRI or X-ray. There are a number of structural problems that occur in our bodies over our lifetimes. Not every structural problem has to be associated with permanent pain. Things like rotator cuff tears, disc degeneration, disc "tears," disc bulges, and meniscal tears are all things that can occur gradually through the process of using our bodies as they were intended. Changes happen in our bodies due to general wear and tear. Our bodies change with age, like it or not, but despite similar processes occurring in everyone's bodies not everyone has terrible pain.

In fact, when you look at patients who have had no pain prior to a relatively minor injury who now have symptoms, it's easy to want to blame the problem on the injury. The reality is that most of the time we're walking around with degenerative changes in our bodies and simply don't have uncontrolled inflammation. Therefore, in many cases, an injury causes the inflammation, which leads to the pain. Steroid injections help to stop that cycle of inflammation and restore you to a pain-free state with minimal intervention by using a combination of local anesthetic and steroids in such sites as your joints, tendons sheaths, muscles, and targeted locations in your neck and spine. These injections can decrease the inflammation and help your pain get better.

Many patients ask me, "How long will this injection last?" Well, that's a really good question. Because the truth is, is that depends a lot on what you do to help your recovery, the severity of your injury, and the inflammatory environment in your body.

Sometimes, the tears and degeneration that that have occurred are things that do require surgical intervention. Sometimes those structural changes need to be corrected. Sometimes patients have real changes in their ability to function. Surgery is sometimes required to restore your ability to move freely.

My hope whenever I give a steroid injection is always that that steroid injection will provide long-term benefit. My hope is that I can spare you from surgery whenever possible. I feel surgery works best when a patient has significant changes to their function. I find that if pain exists without some corresponding structural change and change to function (strength, range of motion, etc.) and that pain does not respond to injections, then the pain usually doesn't respond well to surgery either. Who wants to have surgery if it won't relieve the pain they are having?

Nonsteroidal Anti-inflammatory Medications (NSAIDs)

"I don't want to put that stuff in my body, Doc." I hear it all the time. People don't generally like to take medications, which is why I find it particularly perplexing how quickly someone will turn to something like hydrocodone or oxycodone to treat their symptoms when oftentimes, NSAIDs (medications like naproxen [Aleve], ibuprofen [Advil], and meloxicam [Mobic]) can create significant improvements in your pain. These medications decrease inflammation and help the body heal itself.

Taking anti-inflammatory medications on a regular, short-term basis is safe and appropriate for most patients. Patients with cardiovascular disease, gastric ulcers, high blood pressure, kidney disease, a history of gastric bypass, and those who are pregnant should discuss NSAIDs with their doctor before taking them.

If your doctor has suggested an NSAID to manage your condition, I encourage you to try them regularly for one month. Certainly, there are risks associated with long-term use, and an ongoing consideration of the risks and benefits should be discussed with your doctor. Short courses of these medications are unlikely to harm you if you are otherwise healthy, and they are likely to create significant benefit in your experience of your pain.

Nerve-Stabilizing Medications

The most commonly used nerve-stabilizing medications are pregabalin and gabapentin. These are both part of a class of medications called anticonvulsants. These medications are frequently used to control pain that comes from nerves. They can be used for the management of chronic nerve pain, before surgery, and in the period after surgery to help patients improve their experience of pain. These medications can make a big difference in nerve pain where other medications would fail to provide the same benefit.

Sometimes these medications need to be taken on a long-term, regular basis, like in cases of diabetic neuropathy, as long as the symptoms persist. Sometimes, like after shingles or surgery, people will benefit from taking these medications in the short term. These medications can be particularly useful before and after surgery to help decrease any additional pain that might be caused by the particular surgery that you're having and decrease your use of other medications that may not be as safe. They are especially effective after spine surgeries and knee replacement surgeries.

While some of these medications can have side effects, such as weight gain or sleepiness, a lot of times weight gain can be controlled simply by paying more attention to the foods that you're eating. The sleepiness they cause usually gets better with time as your body gets more used to the medications.

Antidepressants

"Doctor, I'm not depressed. Why do you think I need an anti-depressant? I'm in pain!" Antidepressants, especially tricyclic antidepressants (TCAs) and selective serotonin and norepinephrine re-uptake inhibitors (SNRIs), such as duloxetine, can be highly effective at treating nerve pain and chronic pain conditions such as fibromyalgia.

These medications are not the most effective choices to control depression, but they're very good at controlling nerve pain. They are also pretty good at helping you sleep. So, patients who have problems with sleep due to pain often have significantly improved conditions after using these medications. These medications need to be taken regularly. There is really no benefit to taking them on and off.

There are some side effects from these medications. You want to find the lowest effective dose possible. Your doctor should help you adjust these medications to the right dose for you. Don't be tempted to increase the dose too quickly, because you could have an increased chance of side effects.

Opioids

Opioid medications are indicated in certain forms of pain. They are derived from the poppy plant, just like heroin and opium. These medications are potent pain relievers that also have risky side effects. There are a lot of forms of pain that they don't work well for.

The pain that opiate medications are most helpful to treat is the early stage after a surgical intervention or injury. Sometimes patients are in so much pain right after they're injured that while they're waiting for their injury to be evaluated fully with imaging studies, they would benefit from a short course of a medication like hydrocodone in addition to anti-inflammatory medications and muscle relaxants. These medications can work to supplement other pain relievers. This may improve your symptoms and make it easier for you to function. This is good if it's provoking you to move more freely but not as good if you're becoming reliant on the medication on a regular basis to feel better.

When I discuss opioids with patients who are taking them, they commonly describe their response like this: "It helps for a little while, like an hour or two. Really, I think that it just makes me more able to tolerate the pain for some reason. My pain is still there."

This makes sense because the action of the hydrocodone on the opiate receptors in the brain can release serotonin, which creates a really good feeling. This is why these medications can become so addictive so quickly. People want to feel good, our quest in life is to feel better. Everything that we do is aimed towards feeling better. Whether it be losing weight, getting into a new relationship, having children, or advancing in your career, we focus on our goals because it makes us *feel good*. If there's a medication that we can take that does that job for us, it's awfully easy to get reliant on that medication to do the things that our mind could be doing for itself. It's easier to take a pill than to do the work it takes to feel better.

Opioids are best suited for no more than the first six weeks after an injury or surgical intervention. If you're requiring these medications longer than that you might want to talk to your doctor or pain specialist about trying another, non-opioid medication that might be more effective for the pain that you're having. This takes a person knowledgeable in the treatment of pain and the different types of pain that can occur during the recovery from an injury.

The increasing regulations on opioid use exist because these medications are dangerous, and there is no evidence that they provide any long-term benefit to patients suffering from pain.

I urge you to talk to your specialist about the best combination of medication to treat your pain today.

Radiofrequency Ablation

Sometimes nerves in our body can go haywire. They simply stop sending the messages that they're intended to send. This happens in the spine at the lumbar facet joints when they become arthritic or strained. It also happens at the intercostal nerves (the nerves between your ribs that radiate across from your back to your front) when they might get injured after a strain or fracture or during surgical intervention such as thoracotomy for lung surgery. It can occur at the greater occipital nerve, creating severe headaches that radiate over the top of the head. It can occur at the time of an amputation. When small neuromas form, they can create unbelievable pain.

Many of these nerve targets that are sending inappropriate messages can be easily found using ultrasound and isolated with diagnostic procedures with local anesthetic and can be addressed with more permanent ablative procedures. Sometimes these ablative procedures are surgical in nature. Sometimes the application of heat in the form of radio frequency energy will interrupt these messages. A lot of times these procedures are long lasting but still temporary, meaning that you might see benefits for six months to a year and even sometimes as many as two to five years. However, you may need these procedures repeated in the future. Don't be alarmed by phrases like "burn the nerves," which are often used colloquially to describe the procedure; these procedures are very safe, easily performed, and highly effective in patients who have experienced relief from their pain with temporary local anesthetic diagnostic blocks.

Radiofrequency ablation offers an amazing minimally invasive option for patients who have severe pain from some structures.

Neuromodulation

Neuromodulation can be exceptionally life changing for patients who suffer from long-lasting pain due to complex regional pain syndrome, failed back surgery syndrome, angina, diabetic neuropathy, seizure disorders, peripheral nerve pain, or vascular claudication, among other diagnoses.

What exactly is neuromodulation? Neuromodulation is the process by which small leads are implanted near specific locations that control the pain processing in our body.

These devices can include dorsal root ganglion stimulators, deep brain stimulators, spinal cord stimulators, or peripheral nerve stimulators. All these options involve the implantation of small leads adjacent to easily located structures that are involved in processing your pain. These devices send electrical signals that interrupt the ability of the brain to process sensations as pain. These small electrical signals can be changed and varied in strength, frequency, and location to adapt the therapy to your needs with time.

The process of offering neuromodulation to patients first starts with an insurance-mandated psychological examination and updated imaging studies of the area to be targeted for implantation. Then patients have a trial where these leads are placed at the target area of your pain, and you are connected to an external battery generator for approximately one week. You get to try the therapy before you make any permanent commitment to it.

After a week, the leads are removed. During the week-long trial, you're able to participate in all your usual activities like work and sports, provided you're not bending and twisting too much.

When you return to your doctor, if you've had amazing pain relief, then you can make a choice to implant the device permanently. The implant procedure itself is only a little bit more involved than the trial. Similar leads are placed through a small incision in the skin using the same type of needle that was used for the temporary implant; then the leads are connected to a small battery that's similar in size and design to a pacemaker.

There are a lot of different companies on the market offering these therapies, and while all of them work well for patients, they all offer slightly different options.

If you're interested in trying neuromodulation, consider discussing it with your doctor, preferably a trained interventional pain management specialist who can advise you on the company and therapy that's right for your condition.

I have seen patients do very well with spinal cord stimulation, a form of neuromodulation. Spinal cord stimulation has the potential to improve your function, reduce your need for medication, and improve your quality of life. The results are remarkable—I have even seen patients who were unable to walk without a cane resume walking half a mile at a time just during their trial.

In studies of complex regional pain syndrome, the newest therapy on the market, dorsal root ganglion stimulation, showed 80 percent pain relief on patients who had previously crippling and unrelenting chronic pain from nerve-related pain after surgery. This has been particularly effective in people who have had failed operations to their hips, knees, hernias, and feet, as well as myriad other areas.

Intrathecal Pain Pumps

Intrathecal pain pumps, also known as targeted drug delivery systems, have a tremendous use in patients that have long-standing pain and are reliant on chronic opiate management to control their pain. These conditions are often conditions that are chronic and create pain, things like tumors pressing on nerves, as in cancer patients or patients that have had severe, anatomy-changing injuries, as well as those patients who are limited by side effects from opiate pain management to control their pain.

This device is implanted in the intrathecal space, the space where cerebral spinal fluid is surrounding your spinal cord, and therefore these targeted drug delivery systems provide the medication directly to the cerebral spinal fluid.

I've seen these work wonders in the cancer patients who might have severe constipation or disorientation from the quantity of narcotics that they need to support their pain control. I have also used medications that are nonnarcotic such as ziconitide, a nerve-stabilizing medication that's isolated from snail venom, on patients who have severe chronic neuropathic pain from prior back surgeries or severe traumatic injuries. Talk to your doctor to see if targeted drug delivery may be the right choice for you if you're having side effects from your medications or feel that you need chronic opiate medications in order to manage your ongoing pain.

As you can see, there are lots of different medications that can help create improvements in your pain. I hope you use this information to help and drive discussion with your doctor as you create your treatment plan moving forward.

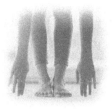

Chapter 11

Obstacles Are Inevitable

As you continue toward improved management of your pain, you will likely encounter many obstacles. You may question your resolve and motivation. You may question the success of the plan. You may question the quality of the treatment from your health care provider.

Of course, there's always a role for a second opinion in the care and management of any health and health condition.

However, consider that sometimes pain is a manifestation and summation of multiple challenges that our body and mind is facing.

Let's discuss some of the obstacles that you may face on your journey.

These Medications Aren't Working

Multiple medications can be prescribed for the management of chronic pain conditions. If you are prescribed a combination of medications and you're finding that they're not successful or not working, I recommend an open dialog with your doctor. Confirm that your doctor is a specialist that is specifically trained in the management of pain conditions. These physicians are usually anesthesiologists or physical medicine and rehabilitation specialists who have devoted extra time in training (a clinical fellowship) to gain knowledge and experience in the treatment of patients suffering from pain. A specialist can advise you on the appropriate combination of medications to address your pain. Not every medication is suited for every specific type of pain condition.

If you feel that a medication that is important to the management of your pain is being withheld from you, consider reviewing some of the strategies in this book. The mindfulness and mindset sections can help you work through these thoughts. When you start feeling negative thoughts about the treatments that you have been offered, those treatments in themselves become less effective. You are stronger than any medication that can be offered to you.

Some medications, such as opiate medications, are associated with worsening pain when taken at escalating dosages. This phenomenon is called "opioid induced hyperalgesia." Sometimes we find that increasing the doses of these medications serves to paradoxically increase the experience of pain rather than decrease it. It doesn't make any sense to continue or increase a pain medication if it may actually function to increase your pain. Think about all the other medications for health conditions that you or your loved ones might take in life, those for diabetes or high blood pressure. If these medications raised your blood sugar or blood pressure, you would never encourage your loved one to increase, let alone continue, the medications. You would advocate for them to fine better alternatives for their care.

When one of my patients, Rachel, first saw me in my office, she was taking remarkably high doses of opioid medications. She alternated between 40 mg long-acting oxycodone three times per day, and 10 mg oxycodone—six to eight additional pills per day! This is equivalent to taking 300 mg of morphine every day! I proposed the idea of "opioid induced hyperalgesia" to her, and she was skeptical at first. However, as she gradually reduced her dosages, she noticed that, remarkably, her pain was actually improving with every pill she discontinued. Now Rachel doesn't rely on opiates to control her pain anymore. Instead, she has increased her activity and notices that a close eye on her diet has the biggest impact on control of her pain. She does occasionally take some medication for her worst days but notices that she needs that extra support only one to two times per week.

Even she is shocked at how much her life has improved after working to reduce her pain pills.

If you had a condition such as high blood pressure and you were taking a medication at escalating dosages month after month and were seeing no change in your blood pressure, you might question if there were other medications that would better suit you to manage this condition, and you would go to a specialist such as a cardiologist and seek other therapies. I encourage you to do the same with your pain medications. If they're not serving you and creating marked and long-lasting improvements in your pain, you need to work to eliminate them.

I Am Afraid of Being Reinjured or I Am Afraid of Injuring Someone Else

Are you afraid of injuring yourself again? Are you afraid of a coworker being injured if you can't fully perform to your capabilities? Are you afraid you aren't functionally able to perform your job as you were previously?

Communication with your physician is very important here. Is your doctor aware of how you feel? Have you fully healed from your injury?

If you have fully healed, then I would suggest that you consider what may be at the root of your fears. Are you still performing the same duties that led to your injury? Perhaps a change in assignment could help. Are your fears a sign of other thoughts? Reflect on the thoughts that drive your emotion of fear.

Create reasonable expectations on your return to work. Perhaps you could ease back in to work, if you have been off a while. You could work with your doctor about limiting your duty hours for the first few weeks back. Talk to your doctor about the limitations you might feel.

If you are fully healed from your condition, the likelihood of reinjury is probably low. Be patient with yourself. Because physically, if you've been out of the game for a few weeks, months, or even years, it might take time to recondition your body to regular constant work.

Even those at desk jobs may find the attention span needed to work through an eight-hour day needs to be retrained if you've been out of work for a period of time. Sometimes the interpersonal relationships at work are exhausting to manage when you've had time alone in your home during your recovery.

Consider the specific thoughts behind your fears.

One patient of mine, Jeff, injured his neck while changing the tire on his car when the jack suspending the car broke and the car nearly crushed him. Quick to move out of the way, he strained his neck and required epidural injections to control his symptoms. He was a laborer in a warehouse and frequently operated pallet jacks in his job duties. While he was recovering, he could not perform the duties of his job due to his physical limitations. When he had recovered from his injuries, he returned to the warehouse. Despite no sign of any cause for pain, he experienced the return of his painful symptoms and experienced panic attacks at work when he returned. He couldn't make it through the workday, and he was at risk of losing everything. He contemplated pursuing disability. When he discussed this with me, I encouraged him to first start doing some work with a therapist and initiate an antidepressant. It turns out that Jeff was suffering from PTSD after his accident, and the pallet jacks were reminding him of the tire jack that had nearly killed him. Adequate treatment of the PTSD resolved his pain symptoms and his panic attacks and allowed him to return to his work without needing to pursue disability.

My Doctor Wants to Wean Me Off These Pain Medications, but They're the Only Thing That I Have

This is a thought that comes up frequently in my practice, especially with the implementation of the new CDC guidelines for physicians in terms of prescribing opiate medications. As opiate medications in some states have become harder and harder to access through one's primary care physician, I've seen patients who've been managed for mild to moderate pain with high doses of opiate medications on a regular basis transferred to myself and my colleagues. These patients arrive perplexed when I discuss the possibility of decreasing their medication that doesn't serve them.

Consider that the health effects of opiates extend widely. Not only do these medications put you at risk for constipation, urinary retention, and sexual dysfunction, but they also create hormonal changes in your body that increase your impulse to consume sweets and increase your risk for diabetes. There are many hormonal impacts of opiate medications that are linked to increased risk of depression and decreased motivation.

If your physician feels that these medications are not an effective tool in your diagnosis of pain, I urge you to keep an open mind. I urge you to consider the possibilities of what your life might look like free from those medications. I have seen many, many patients come off long-term opiate medications and create a dramatically improved outlook on life and in their relationships. This is a similar process to other difficult experiences, such as combating alcoholism.

Improvements in a person's well-being are often associated with some sacrifices, discomfort, and work along the way. The process and the strength that you achieve by overcoming your dependence on these medications, is an important process.

I see over and over again patients coming off these medications and having improvements in their relationships and general sense of well-being. Many go on to create a more positive outlook on life and find new venues for enjoyment in their lives and with their families.

With a strategic approach, no matter how high the dosage of medication is, or regardless of how much you feel that your body requires these medications. I feel strongly that many people can find a better way to manage their pain.

No matter what obstacle you may reach in the pursuit of improved pain, with a strategic approach employing the steps that were outlined in this book, you will be able to conquer your fears and improve your mindset. Every step toward a healthier you is a step toward progress.

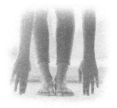

Chapter 12

Team Up

It is impossible to set out on a process such as controlling your pain without an integrated support system behind you. The support system should involve a team of your closest friends, family members, and a strong physician or coach who can lead you through the steps to keep you on your chosen course.

People who achieved dramatic success in life almost invariably have a coach who leads them toward their goals. That coach is not there to police them or to supervise them; they are there as a cheerleader, celebrating their progress along the way and managing obstacles that may be faced. It is important to find a support system that helps keep you on the track toward your goals.

If your goal is to go back to work, move more freely, and find a more inspired and fulfilling existence, despite your pain, then make sure that your doctors and support system are in keeping with that goal.

If you find that your doctor is continually forcing medications on you that you feel do not serve you, have a frank discussion with him or her. And if needed, find another doctor who will help support your well-being.

Most physicians are creatures of their own habits. If their habit is to treat pain only with interventions or with strong medications, then it's hard for them to create different treatment protocols.

There are many physicians to choose from that are motivated and inspired by creating more positive impacts on the life of their patients than medications alone can provide. This is my passion.

Find a doctor who will listen to you and support you. Find someone who will help inspire you to be the person that you most wish to be.

I encourage you to find a physician who has specialty training in pain management and understands fully the risks and benefits of the medications and therapies that may be provided. Your physician should be knowledgeable in the wide range of therapies that are available to treat chronic complex pain conditions.

Strive for improvements, not the elimination of pain. Strive for the improvement of your experience and improvements in your functional abilities even if some pain persists.

Has your physician prescribed physical therapy or advised you on exercise to help encourage your body to toward free movement? Has your physician offered you ideas for nutritional changes that you can make to change your ability and perception of pain?

All of these are important aspects to the comprehensive management chronic pain or a pain that continues after injury or surgery.

You deserve the best physician possible to treat your condition. Keep an open mind and don't pursue someone who only gives you what you want; choose instead someone who strives to make you better.

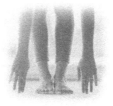

Chapter 13

You Are Stronger
Than Your Pain

We all want one thing in life: freedom. For ages, men and women alike have fought for freedom. The personal war you fight is for the pursuit of freedom of movement and the freedom to pursue the things that create joy in your life. Just as our founding fathers fought for our essential liberties, you must fight to regain your freedom of movement.

Chronic pain can limit your freedom, but you are stronger than the pain that holds you back. Your pain is just a circumstance. You can change that circumstance with simple changes in your approach to your pain that create powerful influence over your emotions.

Change your mindset today toward a healthier life and you will see your circumstances shift. Freedom from pain cannot be accomplished in a day, a week, or a month. Your path forward will be made with continual and constant redirection toward the simple steps of mindfulness, fueling your body with nutritious, anti-inflammatory food, becoming more aware of your thought patterns, and regular exercise. These things, in combination with medications, interventions, and supplements will help and provide you the most pain free state possible.

I have introduced you to patients of mine who have conquered unbelievable levels of pain. I have shown you how my patients create miracles in their lives. I have seen patients who thought the quest for improvement was hopeless find an entirely new outlook on life just by implementing some of these simple steps on a regular basis and following a targeted treatment plan to manage their pain.

You are capable of implementing this process in your life. While this process may not eliminate your pain, I know that when you work the steps of this process that you will find unbelievable improvements in your abilities to manage the pain you experience. You will suffer less. These steps will likely improve all aspects of your life, not just your pain, but also your relationships, your employment, and your family life.

There is no reason to suffer helplessly in pain. We were given the gift of life to enjoy.

The processes outlined in this book will lead you toward better control over your circumstances and an improved outlook. You will move freely again.

Acknowledgments

I could never write this book without the opportunity to care for the patients who I love so much. My passion for the field of Interventional Pain Management drives me continually forward to seek the best possible options of care for my patients. At some point, the cutting-edge treatments that we practice and perfect are simply not enough to create change. This book was born out of my continual drive to want better lives for my patients.

Each of my patients has taught me the skills that allow me to perfect my practice and grow in my knowledge. This book is the product of countless conversations about the inner drive and motivation of the patient suffering from pain and their commitment to improving their lives. Thank you for sharing your stories with me.

With all of the commitments of my full-time practice, this book would not be possible without the commitment of my staff to my vision of patient-centered care. My staff members, who each love my patients as I do, help me to care for each individual by being always willing to support, empathize, and listen to the challenges and fears my patients face in the management of their pain. There would be no way for me to effectively share my message without the excellent support system I have in my practice.

To Margie, my medical assistant, your instinct and attention to detail are unparalleled. I appreciate your loyalty as we grow. I am grateful for all that you do to support me and my patients. To Debby, my office manager, you are the glue that keeps the details together. Your leadership has created a cohesive group of women devoted to patient care. Vicky, Maulinda, Terri, and Shelly my patients appreciate the smiles on your faces and the welcoming environment you create when scheduling patients, greeting them at the door, and addressing their questions on the phone. You help me create a space where patients can heal.

To the Morgan James Publishing team: Special thanks to David Hancock, CEO & Founder for believing in me and my message. To my Author Relations Manager, Margo Toulouse thanks for making the process seamless and easy. Many more thanks to everyone else, but especially Jim Howard, Bethany Marshall, and Nickcole Watkins.

To Krystina and Kim, you are the best teammates, and friends, that a doctor could have. You helped refine a process for patient care that is patient centered and efficient. I may not get to keep you with me all the time, but I cherish the days that we share.

To Matt, you always believe in me and challenge me to be my best. You are my mentor, and I appreciate the knowledge you share with me. I still have so much to learn from you.

No book can be created without a strong editorial team. Thank you, Moriah, for keeping me on track. I know that I have a lot of plates spinning in the air and that I am hard to keep up with sometimes - but thank you for your faith in me. Angela, thank you for the entire process that helped me direct my attention toward moving forward to write this book. You inspire me more than you could possibly know.

Kristen, you have been there for me since the beginning. Thank you for always looking out for the best for me and showing me perspectives I haven't considered.

Shawn, my everything, you always encourage me to pursue my dreams. Thank you for waking up with me every day, taking such good care of our little girls, and picking up the shoes I leave by the door. I am grateful for the time and space you give me to grow in my career.

To Nora and Bridget, you made me a mom, and I hope that I can inspire you to live a life invested in sharing your message with the world and improving others' lives with your kindness.

Finally, to my parents. Without you, none of my accomplishments would have ever been possible. You are the voices in my head that compel me forward.

I love you all.

About the Author

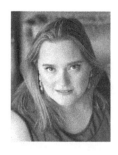

Helen M. Blake, MD is a Board Certified Anesthesiologist and Board Certified Pain Management specialist. She has devoted her career to helping patients manage the pain that limits them. Dr. Blake specializes in the care of patients who have been injured at work or in motor vehicle accidents and helps them reclaim their lives after facing unexpected challenges. She has devoted the past six years of her practice at Pain and Rehabilitation Specialists of Saint Louis to the comprehensive care of her patients and stays current in the most novel of therapies. She is active in clinical research, an expert consultant to industry, and active in her professional societies.

Dr. Blake had the privilege to train at some of the nation's most respected specialty hospitals including the Hospital for Special Surgery, Weill Cornell Medical Center, and Memorial Sloan Kettering Cancer Center. She graduated from Saint Louis University Medical School with Distinction in Research after collaboration on research projects with the National Cancer Institute, National Institutes of Health. She was awarded membership in the Alpha Sigma Nu honor society for her scholarship, loyalty, and service to Saint Louis University. Dr. Blake is a Langsdorf Fellow alumnus of Washington University in Saint Louis and was awarded a full scholarship for her academic achievements.

Dr. Blake is devoted to her family. When she is not working, she enjoys the peace of the outdoors. Even though she has settled in the Midwest, she tries to be near the water every chance she can.

Thank You!

I am grateful that you took the time to read my book!

If you would like to learn more tips from me about managing your pain and moving freely stop by my website at www.liveandmovefreely.com and sign up for my newsletter.

I would love to hear from you and connect with you! Feel free to find me, Helen M. Blake, MD on my Facebook page. Be sure to like it to follow all the great things happening in my medical practice.

I am currently accepting new patients. You can find my practice at www.prsstl.com. Whether your injury was six months or six years ago, I can help you get the results that you need to manage your pain.

I can't wait to help you move freely.

CPSIA information can be obtained
at www.ICGtesting.com
Printed in the USA
BVHW031102121119
563577BV00001B/95/P

9 781642 794588